Lyn and Me
Our life with MS and beyond

Roger Hammond

foreword by Professor John Greenwood

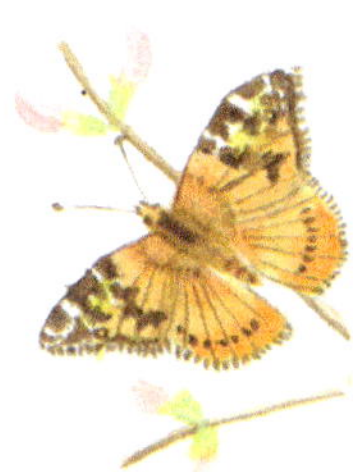

Lyn and Me Our life with MS and beyond
by
Roger Hammond

ISBN: 978-1-7395589-6-3

Published by Exmoor News www.exmoornews.co.uk

EXMOOR NEWS

Roger Hammond has lived in Dulverton on Exmoor since 2010, having moved there from Harrow Weald, North West London. He is an architectural designer and artist, with a keen interest in photography. Roger and his wife, Lyn, had wanted to move to the West Country for some time; they were thinking of future retirement and, having visited the area frequently over the years, it was an obvious choice. Lyn, who had been diagnosed with primary progressive multiple sclerosis in 1995, also needed to move into a single-storey home to make things easier—and to be within walking or scooter distance of a small town. Dulverton fitted the bill on all counts. Roger took up writing in 2022, following the passing of his beloved wife, Lyn, as he wanted to create a fundraising legacy in her name.

In loving memory of Linda Anne Hammond (Lyn), a much loved and much missed wife, mother, grandmother (Nana) and friend to many.

Sadly, Lyn's much loved brother, Neil, passed away five days after her, leaving his lovely wife, Pik Lin, so this book also honours his memory.

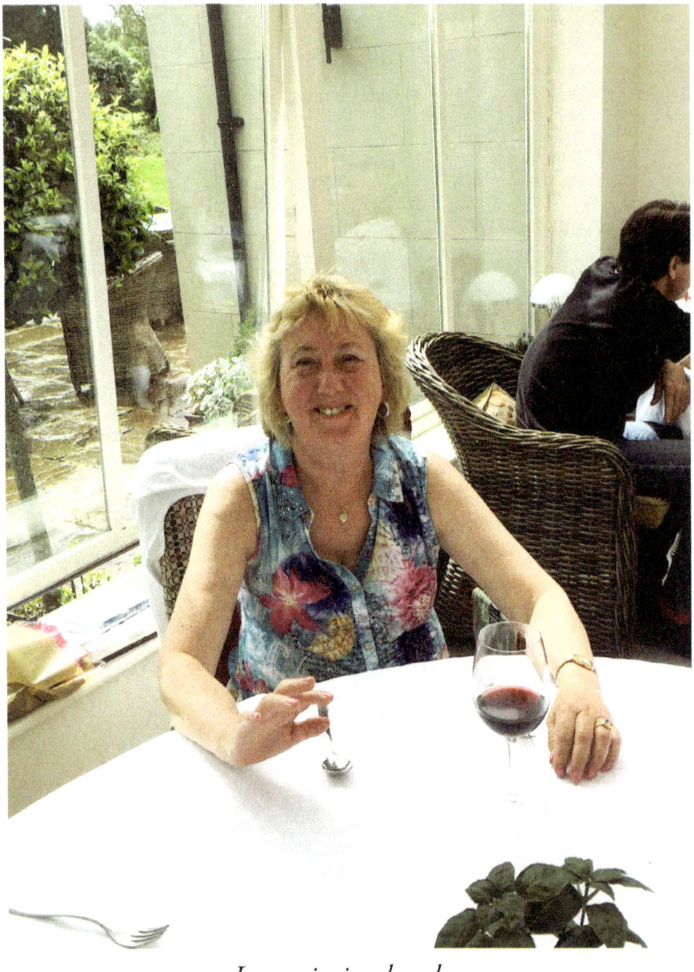

Lyn enjoying lunch.

Foreword

There have been many moving first-hand accounts written by individuals affected by debilitating disease, including that of Multiple Sclerosis (MS). Indeed, these personal stories can provide helpful guidance for those with MS but equally, for those of us not affected, provide insight into the remarkable courage and resilience often exhibited. Rarely, however, do we find written accounts from the unaffected partner—the silent carer—whose life is also changed forever.

This personal account, written by Roger Hammond, whose wife Lyn lived for many years with MS, addresses this gap. It is a deeply touching and poignant description of life from the partner's perspective and is written in an easy conversational style with wonderful honesty and passion. Most important, it shows that, despite the increasing challenges they faced, a rewarding and fulfilling life can still be lived, underpinned by enduring love, deeply shared interests and great humour.

Roger's account also reveals his remarkable resolve in challenging the support system, and in making the most of the limited resources available. Of course, it is not without the inevitable lows and frustrations, but the overwhelming message is one of positivity. His informal and intimate style, from a rarely articulated perspective, is powerful; Roger writes openly about his experience, not in a self-indulgent way, but in an unpretentious and genial manner. It is a book that is both uplifting and valuable as a source of much-needed information for anyone finding themselves in a similar situation.

Professor John Greenwood
University College London

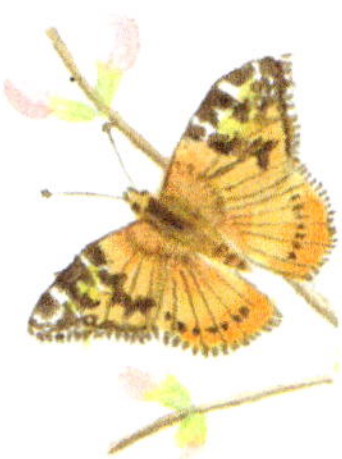

Table of Contents

1 Prologue

When I embarked on the journey of writing this book I did not know where it was going to take me. I had wanted, for some time, to think of something positive I could do in Lyn's memory, a legacy if you will. I seriously thought about the Dart10k open water swim as a fundraiser; it would have attracted plenty of support and raised a fair amount of money.

My head said 'yes' because, physically, the distance would have been fine stamina-wise as I have always been a distance swimmer. But my heart had to say 'no'; I have a heart condition and was advised not to swim in very cold open water, even with a wet suit, so that was a non-starter.

I did think of other fundraising ideas but then rejected them.

Some months after Lyn passed away, I was sitting watching what I can only describe as some mindless TV programme one evening, glass of wine in hand. I was thinking of writing something, but what? A possible title suddenly hit me: My Life with MS, a husband's perspective.

I have always had a pen and paper near me; I am forever making notes for myself. After the title, I wrote two sides of A4 paper, with chapter headings, in a matter of minutes—without much thought. I think Lyn was up there guiding me to do this, otherwise it would not have come so easily.

Lyn and I were married for forty-seven years, and I was her carer for thirty of those years. This book is not intended to sanctify Lyn, nor to make myself look good for the help that I willingly and lovingly gave her during the years I was caring for her, but as our story. It started life as a self-help book, maybe for someone newly diagnosed with multiple sclerosis (MS) and unsure about anything, or maybe for someone who is now a carer and does not necessarily know much about the role. That is how it started but the process of writing has taken on a life of its own; it is now a cross between a self-help book, a biography and a love story. Not a bad mix—it is what it is.

So this was us. It is what our life was like with MS and beyond; our life story, no holds barred, warts and all and, hopefully, a better understanding for those who follow me on the journey.

As there are variations in forms of address and how people identify these days—and I do want to include all possible variations whenever I am referring to someone in a relationship—I will simplify my version here. Lyn was my wife and she is referred to as that. I will use spouse to mean either someone who is married or a partner in a relationship. Life carer means just that.

I have used extracts in this book from the MS Society's website and other organisations, which are acknowledged and credited as such.

This does not read like a conventional biography as it does not follow a strict timeline; it unfolds to suit the content, so bear with me.

2 Multiple Sclerosis

You cannot die from MS. You may die from complications, from something else during a hospital admission for an unrelated condition such as pneumonia, or anything else that may come in unexpectedly from the side. (I am not a doctor; I have no medical qualifications and anything I may say in this book is based solely on personal experience.)

There are four types of MS, the MS Society produces a booklet entitled *Types of MS*; here is an extract from their website:

> Benign MS, Relapsing remitting MS (RRMS) Primary progressive MS (PPMS) and Secondary progressive MS (SPMS).
>
> Benign MS:
> The term Benign MS is sometimes used to describe a version of relapsing remitting MS with very mild or no attacks separated by long periods with no symptoms. 'Benign' means 'something doesn't cause any harm'. You can only really say you have benign MS after you've gone 15 years or so without many symptoms and you've got little or no disability. A diagnosis of benign MS doesn't guarantee you'll be free of symptoms.
> You might still get things like fatigue or problems with your memory or thinking.
> MRI scans can still show MS is damaging your

brain and spinal chord even if yours seems mild. After many years of your MS appearing to be 'benign' it's possible you might have a relapse. The term isn't recommended as it can only describe your past experience of MS, not whether you might relapse in the future.

Relapsing remitting MS (RRMS):

In relapsing remitting MS (RRMS) people have attacks of new and old symptoms, this is called a relapse. Around 85% of people with multiple sclerosis are diagnosed with RRMS. Taking a disease modifying therapy (DMT) could mean fewer relapses and slow down your MS.

The relapsing remitting label can help to explain MS to others and help you to find the best treatments. But it can't predict exactly how MS will affect you. For most people with MS, this is the way their MS begins, except for the small group of people (15%) diagnosed with primary progressive MS.

Relapsing remitting MS is a type of MS where you have relapses (symptoms getting worse) followed by recovery (that's when it's "remitting").

Relapsing-remitting MS is generally marked by relapses that last at least 24 hours. During a relapse, the symptoms may get worse. Common symptoms of RRMS include one or more of the following: Sensitivity to heat. Difficulty seeing or vision problems. Fatigue. Muscle weakness. Numbness, particularly in the feet. During a relapse, the symptoms may get worse.

Primary progressive MS;

Primary progressive MS (PPMS) is called this because from the first, or primary, symptoms it's progressive. It's usually diagnosed in people in their 40s.

Early symptoms are often subtle, like problems with walking, which develop over time. There will usually be few or no relapses with PPMS. Instead, disability will gradually increase. There can also be long periods where symptoms seem to be staying level.

People with primary progressive MS can experience many of the same symptoms as those with relapsing remitting MS.

To get a diagnosis of primary progressive MS you must have had no remissions or relapses, but your disability must have got worse over at least a year. An MRI scan must show two or more lesions in different parts of your brain or spinal cord. These must have happened at different times. A lumbar puncture must also show signs of MS (antibodies) in the fluid around your spinal cord.

Some people also get relapses early on in primary progressive MS, or their scans show inflammation in the shape of new lesions. This is called active primary progressive MS (it used to be called 'progressive relapsing MS').

'Active' here means the person's immune system is still attacking the myelin around nerves in their brain or spinal chord, and causing inflammation. A relapse or new lesions on MRI scans are signs of this.

Secondary progressive MS;

Secondary progressive multiple sclerosis (SPMS) is characterized by gradual worsening of disability. Symptoms of SPMS include fatigue, numbness or tingling, vision problems, spasticity or stiffness of the muscles, bowel and bladder problems, and problems with cognition. Other symptoms that might indicate a shift to SPMS include severe weakness or paralysis, muscle stiffness or spasms, mood problems, and sexual dysfunction.

What is well known is that the immune system is your body's defence against infection. In MS, the immune system treats the protective myelin coating around nerves like an infection. This leads to myelin being destroyed.

Myelin plays a really important role in making sure messages can be sent from the brain to the rest of the body efficiently, as well as protecting the nerve from damage. So when myelin is damaged, the nerve stops working properly. We don't yet know exactly why the immune system attacks myelin in MS.

What causes MS

MS is not directly inherited from parent to child. There's no single gene that causes it. Over 200 genes might affect your chances of getting MS. But genes are only part of the story.

MS can happen more than once in a family, but it's much more likely this will not happen.

There's only about a 1.5% chance of a child developing MS when their mother or father has it (that means around 1 in 67 get it). There's only around a 2.7% chance that you'll get MS if your brother or sister has it (around 1 in 37). In 2014 a very large study found that MS may be even less likely to be passed on than these figures suggest. You're not born with symptoms of MS.

If you develop MS it's usually diagnosed in your 30s or 40s. However it can also develop earlier or later than that. There's currently no way to tell whether someone will develop MS later in life.

What happens to myelin in MS

Nerve cells carry messages between the brain and spinal chord and the organs and limbs of the body. They control everything we do – from how we move to how we think and feel.

Myelin is the fatty protective coating that surrounds nerve fibres – a bit like the insulation on an electrical wire. As well as protecting the fragile nerve fibres, myelin also allows messages to travel quickly along the nerves without being lost or interrupted.

For example, in the nerve cells that extend from the spinal chord to the muscle in your leg, the myelin coating allows messages to travel at up to 268 miles per hour. In nerve cells without myelin, the speed of the message travels at can drop as low as 1 mile per hour.

The above are all extracts from the MS Society website, which offers more detail about the various types; you can find more information in the bibliography at the end of this book.

In simple terms the Myelin Sheath is the "protective insulation" around the nerves in the body. Imagine an electrical cable: it has copper wiring inside, with an insulation layer outside that stops any damage to the wiring inside. If the outer insulation of an electrical cable is damaged, it can cause short circuits and lead to any number of problems.

In MS, the myelin sheath is the insulation that breaks down; the nerve signals from the brain to various parts of the body are scrambled and do not work properly.

Disease modifying therapies are available; there is plenty of information about them on the MS Society website:

Disease modifying therapies (DMTs) aren't a cure for MS, but they can reduce how many relapses someone has and how serious they are. They can also slow down the damage caused by MS that builds up over time.

Disease Modifying Therapies (DMTs) are treatments that could change (for the better) how your MS develops over time.

A DMT could be a drug you take. Sometimes you'll hear them called 'disease modifying drugs' (DMDs). A DMT could also be a treatment that uses stem cells. A DMT isn't a cure, but it could make a real difference to your MS. These treatments can offer many people the chance to take more control of their MS.

There are over a dozen DMTs for MS available on the

NHS. They're taken either as a pill, an injection or an infusion.

Our DMT decision tool is here to help you explore your DMT options and prepare for conversations with health professionals.

If you are newly diagnosed, it would be worth looking at the MS Society website information about your particular type, as well as talking to your health professionals, consultants, doctors and specialist nurses, as it will give you a more in-depth explanation. Having information at your fingertips is essential to a greater understanding of what you are dealing with and it is always there for you to go over or refresh your memory.

3 Early life

Lyn was born on 14 May 1953 at Bushey Maternity Hospital. Her mum, Margaret (Morgan), was Welsh, born in Llanelli, South Wales; she had moved to England in the late 1940s looking for work and following her sister, Gwen, who had moved to England earlier and, coincidentally, had married her dad Derek's uncle Dick.

Derek and Margaret married in January 1952, and they lived for many happy years in Harrow. They had three children, Lyn (Linda), Neil and Peter, and a happy life, first in Carmelite Road and later in a house in Maricas Avenue, Harrow Weald.

Unfortunately, Margaret developed breast cancer and passed away in early 1971 when Lyn was eighteen, a very vulnerable age for a teenage girl to lose her mum. Neil and Peter were younger, at sixteen and eleven respectively, and they needed a mother figure in their lives. Lyn's paternal grandmother, Amy, lived in Belmont, not that far away by bus and on foot, so she stepped in and was there to deal with all the domestic duties and cooking evening meals, as well as providing some much needed love and support. They were all very lucky to have her help for a few years.

Lyn's dad had always worked night shifts for Post Office Telephones, as it was called before the BT brand, so it was difficult for him to be at home all the time. In 1972, Derek married Vi; they had both worked for Post Office Telephones and had known each other for some years. They continued to live in Maricas Avenue for the rest of their lives; Derek passed away in 2007, followed by Vi in 2017. They were loving grandparents to our daughters, Sarah and Kelly, and Peter's children, Christian, Amy and Elliott.

Growing up, Lyn was just a normal healthy girl; the only major setback she had as a child was a depressed sternum, as had her brother, Neil. When she was very young, Lyn had a largely successful operation to correct this. They all had the normal childhood illnesses and bugs but nothing out of the ordinary.

I was born on 2 September 1952 at Edgware General Hospital. My mum, Winnie, and dad, Arthur, both lived and met in College Road, Harrow Weald, and were married in 1949. After they married, my mum and dad lived with me in Wealdstone until after my brother Keith was born on 9 January 1955. We moved to Stanmore when I was five and then to College Road, Harrow Weald when I was twelve. I did not know then that Lyn and I lived just a couple of streets away from each other.

Not only did we live near each other but, not long after I met Lyn, I met her parents Derek and Vi and her brothers, Neil and Peter, and then her grandparents, Harry and Amy. Talking with Harry one day, I told him that my family had lived in Harrow Weald for many years. He asked me what my grandfather's name was; when I told him, he said he used to work with an Arthur Hammond at the Post Office engineering department in the 1930s. That was quite a coincidence but, bearing in mind that the greater Harrow area was a very small place in the 1920s to '40s, it was not unusual that our grandfathers would have known each other.

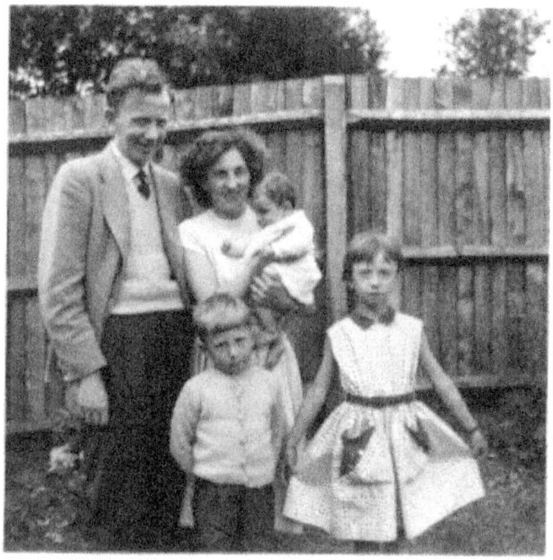

Lyn's dad and mum, with baby Peter, Neil and Lyn.

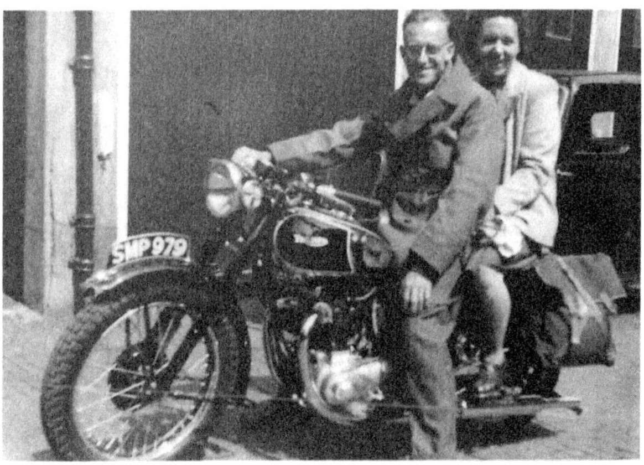

My parents.

4 Meeting Lyn

I met Lyn in 1971, by gatecrashing a party, after a fashion; I was already nineteen and she had just turned nineteen. At that time, a group of friends and I would meet at a pub on a Friday evening, either The Railway Tavern in Hatch End or The Victory in Pinner, for a few beers.

It was quite normal for someone to say, 'There's a party in Paddington on Saturday. Does anyone fancy going?' Silly question to ask a group of nineteen-year-old lads, really…

In this case, a friend of mine, Alan knew a girl named Lyn, whose friend, Chrissie, was sharing a flat with two other girls and they were having the party.

So, on that Saturday we all made our way down to Paddington, bought some beers on the way—might even have been a Party Seven, an enormous seven-pint can of beer, very popular for parties at the time. We found the address and knocked on the door.

'Hi, John invited us.' There was always someone named John at any party, so it was the standard opening line.

'Oh right, yeah, come in.'

In we went, put the beers in the kitchen, grabbed one each, and started mingling.

I do not remember anything much about the party that evening but I do remember going out to the garden at some point—probably for a cigarette, as I did smoke back then. (I gave up thirty-five years or so ago.) As I wandered around, I noticed a girl sitting on a bench on her own. The exact words are lost in the mists of time, but they went something like this:

'Are you OK?' I asked.

'Yes, I'm OK. No…not really.'

'Mind if I sit down?'

"Yes, it's OK.'

'I'm Roger.'

'Lyn.'

'So, why are you out here on your own?'

'I just needed some space.'

'Oh, OK, why?'

Lyn then started to talk and, for the most part, I listened. (That rather set the scene for the rest of our lives.) She had lost her mum to breast cancer the previous year, so she was still grieving. Her dad had remarried and she was having a difficult time accepting a stepmother so soon after her mum had passed away. It was causing her much anxiety and confusion—all the emotional issues you would expect from that kind of situation.

We talked about so many things for what seemed like hours. It felt as though she was just opening up to someone, for the first time in ages; we seemed to have clicked and, at some point, we rejoined the party. We resumed socialising—separately—but I made sure that I had her telephone number. We had all stayed the night; I went home with the lads in the morning and went back to the normal life of a nineteen-year-old lad.

I did call Lyn, the first of many calls that led to us keeping in touch, using the public telephone box at the end of my road. For those of you unfamiliar with these, it was a large red box with many glass panes, designed by architect, Sir

Giles Gilbert Scott, who was also responsible for Liverpool Cathedral. This one was located at the end of Long Elms, a road in Harrow Weald, more or less midway between our houses. You opened the telephone kiosk door and went in, and the telephone was there in front of you. It was a black box on the wall with a telephone handset on top; below that was a slot for coins, with a small dish below and some large A and B letters moulded on the face of the box. You lifted the handset and dialled the number; if that was correct, the other party answered—you pressed button A and you were connected. If no-one was there and it carried on ringing, you pressed button B and your money landed back in a small dish. If you never experienced the magic and frustration of this wondrous piece of equipment, you do not know what you missed!

Why did I use a public telephone box? There were no mobile phones back then and the only option was a landline. My mum and dad had a telephone but, to reduce the cost, they shared the line with the next-door neighbours; it was called a party line, something totally alien to anyone now. It was a guessing game back then as to whether your neighbours were on the phone; you picked up the handset to make a call and someone would be talking…so you replaced it and tried again later.

Now, it is so easy to send and receive a few texts in the space of a few minutes and organise your social life for a week or even months ahead. As time went on we started dating; sometimes, I would walk to the end of the road and call Lyn; sometimes, I would go round to see her, or she came round to me. It depended on what we were both doing.

We were both working: I was an architectural designer in Wembley and Lyn was an administrative assistant at the Department of Employment and Social Security in Harlesden, which was better known internally back then as the 'Department of Enjoyment and Promiscuity'...She had met new friends there, including Chrissie, who had moved to London from Nantwich in Cheshire for work, and whose fiancé, Tim, was still studying agriculture at Manchester University. Lyn and Chrissie clicked when they first met and were destined to become lifelong best friends. They also bonded, because they had both lost their mothers to breast cancer. In fact, Chrissie was living with two other girls at the house in Sutherland Avenue, Paddington, where I had first met Lyn.

Before I met her, Lyn had done some modelling and I still have some of the professional photos that were taken at the time.

Our relationship blossomed over a couple of years, and we shared the experience of expanding our circle of friends and enjoyed life, like any young couple. We would meet our friends in one of the many pubs we all used to frequent, went to parties, gigs, and did all the things you normally do when you are going out with someone.

We had an old Ford Popular, Lyn having passed her driving test before me. She had paid £15.00 for it, which sounds like a miniscule amount to spend on a car now but, in 1971 and, at our age, that was a week's wages. What an amazing car it was, a weird kind of mint green colour with a yellow and red 'go-faster' stripe down the sides. We drove it all over the place for several years.

In 1971, we both changed jobs; Lyn became an

administrative assistant at Canon Assurance in Wembley, and I was working as an architectural designer in Whetstone, near Barnet. I sometimes went into London for work, so she would give me a lift to catch the tube at Wembley Park on her way to work.

One morning, we were going up the hill towards Preston Road roundabout and the traffic stopped. Lyn stopped and tried the handbrake but it would not pull up; she started to panic a bit, so I grabbed it and lifted—the handbrake came off in my hand. I sat there holding up the handbrake, with the cable dangling; Lyn looked at me in horror. I looked round and saw the car behind us reversing at a rate of knots as he could see what had happened and what I was holding in my hand…I do not remember how, but we got to the top of the hill and took the car to the garage opposite to get it fixed.

We eventually managed to sell the Ford Popular, which was a quite a surprise but it turned out that the buyer was just interested in the number plate! We then upgraded to a Hillman Super Minx, for which we paid £35.00, the equivalent of two weeks' wages.

A couple of Lyn's friends had boyfriends who were well into their cars and we went to race meets and drag car races at Santa Pod, near Northampton, a few times; the noise, speed and atmosphere were quite addictive.

We went on several trips to stay with friends like Chrissie and Tim, who had married in Nantwich in 1972, and we went away for a week on our first holiday together to Rhyl in North Wales after their wedding.

It was difficult to go away as a couple; you had to hide it from your parents, as they would not have approved, but somehow we managed. It is much more open and easier now, which is a very good thing. Lyn said that her mum had once told her, 'There will always be someone out there for you; you just have to find them.'

I guess that was me.

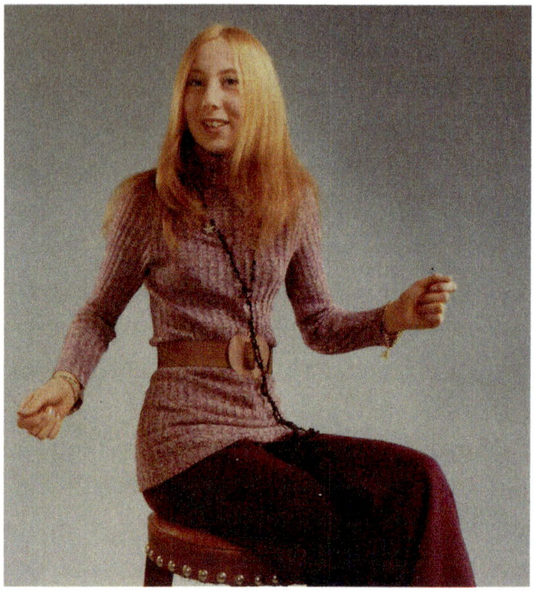

Lyn modelling 1970.

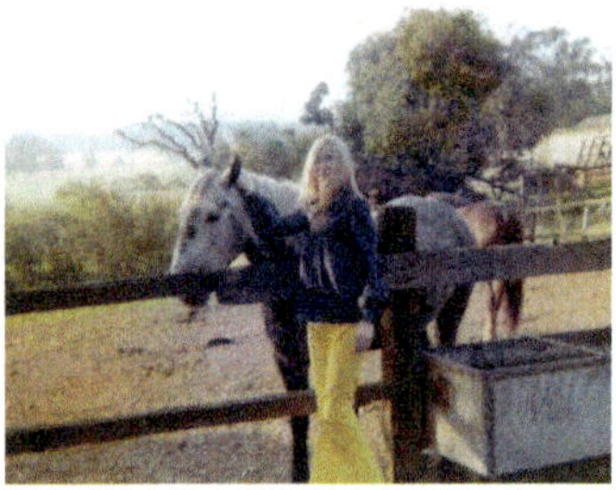

Lyn 1972.

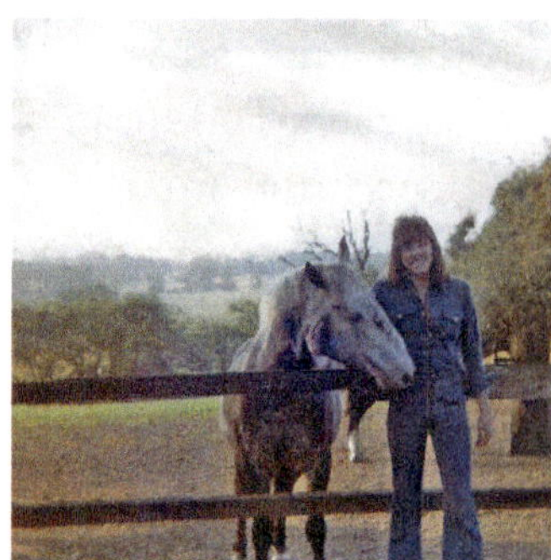

Me 1972.

5 Marriage and the early years

I proposed to Lyn outside the Dirty Duck pub in Stratford-upon-Avon. Of course, she said, 'Yes.' We were there for a long weekend of cultural sightseeing and some fun.

Life went on and we started to talk about what we wanted to do and made plans for our future together, as well as visiting each other's relatives, as everyone did when they became engaged. While she was growing up, Lyn had often spent time visiting her mum's relatives in Llanelli, South Wales, so it was only natural that we went to stay with her cousin, Marlene, and her husband, Jeff, and visited all her other relatives while we were there, the first of many occasions. After a few visits I was 'adopted' by her Welsh family, which led to me supporting Welsh rugby when they played anyone but England.

We married on 28 September 1974 at All Saints' Church, Harrow Weald, where my mum and dad had married in April 1949, so we carried on the tradition.

In those days we could not have afforded a house in Harrow Weald, or anywhere near it, so we moved to Stevenage, Hertfordshire. We had considered quite a few places, but Lyn's cousin, Janice, was living there with her mum, Jean, and stepdad, Peter. This gave us a link to the area, with people we already knew.

Lyn got a job with Stevenage Borough Council doing administrative work; a year later and because of her previous experience, she secured a transfer within the Civil Service to the Land Registry in Stevenage. Everything was falling into place.

We loved our first house; we spent time decorating it, fitting a new kitchen and bathroom, installing a central heating system—with the help of my dad, who could turn his hand to most things—and improving the small garden. We also made some new friends.

I had changed jobs in 1975, as I could not see a future with the firm I was working for; it did not seem to be going anywhere and I needed something positive for my future and to be able to provide for my family. As a stop-gap, I took a job locally; this reduced travel costs and gave me time to look for a post that might lead to a better future.

While working locally, I applied for several jobs and was eventually offered one at a leading property consultancy in London; I grabbed it with both hands. It meant travelling into London, but the salary and prospects far outweighed that.

We lived in Stevenage from 1974 to 1982; it was a very happy time and, around 1977, we decided to start a family. Sarah was born on 16 September 1978 at 1.00pm in Hitchin Hospital. We had been out on that Saturday morning looking for wallpaper and paint, Lyn felt a bit of a twinge in her tummy; we did not take much notice of it, as the due date was still two weeks away. Twenty minutes later, another twinge; maybe something was happening. Then another…we headed home.

Our neighbour, Margaret, thought we were too entirely laid back about the whole thing, sitting in the kitchen having sandwiches and cups tea before we left for the hospital. Margaret pushed us out of the house. We grabbed the pre-packed maternity bag and other items, put everything in the car, and headed to Hitchin Hospital. As soon as we arrived at the hospital's maternity unit, they examined Lyn and said, 'You need to go straight into the delivery suite.'

Sarah was born about fifteen minutes later on a wonderful sunny Saturday afternoon; everything was right in the world. A couple of days later, we went home, got used to our new baby, and slowly but surely got into a routine. It was not easy—as first-time parents, it never is—but we got there.

From the start of our marriage, we had always shared household chores, such as cooking, washing or cleaning. It always just seemed a natural thing to do, so helping with a new baby just came naturally. To give Lyn a break from looking after Sarah during the week, I did the weekend night shift, changing and feeding; one night I got up three times… First, Sarah threw up over my shoulder as I winded her, so I went back to bed minus my T-shirt. Next, Sarah did a wee, so I lost my second T-shirt. And the third time it was a poo, so I lost my pyjama bottoms to the washing basket and trotted back to bed naked, the first of many similar occasions.

Lyn was looking after Sarah all week but, some months later, she decided she needed something to vary the routine and took a Saturday job at a town centre jewellery store. This gave her an outlet, a chance to do something different, meet people, and earn some extra cash, which was important back then. I was quite happy to spend my Saturdays looking after and playing with Sarah, doing chores while she slept.

A couple of years later, we decided to expand our little

family and at Hitchin Hospital, on 2 May 1981—another wonderfully sunny Saturday afternoon, our second daughter, Kelly, was born, I did the night shifts with Kelly, as I had with Sarah, as it gave Lyn a break at the weekends. As all parents know, bringing up a second child is far easier and more relaxed than the first time round.

We now had our ideal family; Lyn was a very good mum, always doing things with the girls, taking them to pre-school playgroups, meeting up with other young mums, and driving to Harrow now and then to take the girls to their grandparents. About this time my dad had bought a new car, so we bought his Vauxhall Viva estate, making life so much easier. Having a more modern and reliable car, with rather more sturdy metal protection, made me feel better when Lyn travelled anywhere with the girls.

It also meant that I did not have to spend what seemed to be a part of every weekend either working in the open bonnet or underneath the car fixing something. I once removed the prop shaft from the Hillman Super Minx, as it needed a new universal joint fitted, and—much to the surprise of the mechanic at the local garage—I wrapped it in paper and took it on the bus to save on the repair costs.

Like many other property owners, we were thinking of improving our property or moving somewhere else, when time and funds allowed. When we decided to move away, we looked at nearby towns, such as Hitchin, Letchworth and Baldock, but could not find anything that worked for us. But, in 1982, we had the mad idea to move away and build our own house… I discovered that Milton Keynes Development Corporation was encouraging people to move into the area, to design their own homes, and to be part of a growing community.

With the help of a loan from my dad to buy the building plot, we started the process. I designed the house, got the planning and building regulations approvals, and, with plenty of help from local tradespeople—and plenty of work from me in the evenings after work and at weekends—we built it in twelve months. We finally finished in 1983 and moved in.

It was great; we enjoyed the house and the area, and were constantly making new friends. Lyn was a social animal and made friends very easily, especially with Sarah starting school, where Lyn met other mums.

However, 1984 started sadly, as my mum passed away in February. She and dad had stayed with us at Christmas and we both knew she was very ill. They had arrived on Christmas Eve but I had not seen my mum for a couple of months and I was shocked to see how frail she had become in such a short time; not at all her normal, bubbly self. She had never mentioned anything to my dad about feeling ill; it was as if it had just crept up on them.

Christmas was very quiet; we did as much as we could with Sarah and Kelly, but we were concerned about my mum, who spent most of the time resting in bed. I called my brother, Keith, and told him what was happening. The day after Boxing Day, I called the emergency doctor from our local surgery; he examined her and said we should get her home as quickly as possible and call her GP. I called my brother and then drove back to Harrow with my mum and dad; we called the doctor, who arranged for her to go to hospital that afternoon. After tests the following day, we all met at the hospital; the consultant told us it was bowel cancer, with secondary liver cancer, and it was terminal. The doctors said she would have about six months; the reality was weeks rather than months. Mum never left hospital and passed away six weeks later, a huge loss to us all.

Later in 1984, we found out that Lyn was pregnant, and we were looking forward to having another baby; it was a bit of a shock at the first scan to learn that she was going to have twins… It was even more of a shock when Lyn had a miscarriage and lost one of the twins at three months; she stayed in hospital for a few days to ensure that everything was fine with her and the other twin. That was bad enough but, three months later, she lost the second twin. We were both devastated.

At three months, yes, you would consider it as a miscarriage, but at six months, although not a viable survival term for a foetus at that time, it felt like a normal birth to Lyn. Understandably, she reacted as if she had lost a full-term baby at birth—pain, sorrow, guilt and anger all together and all at the same time. Forty years ago, there was little support for the mothers in Lyn's situation in the hospital; as the babies were not full term, they were just treated as miscarriages, and you were almost left to get on with it, without any advice, help or support on how to cope with the situation at the time or in the future.

Things have improved over the years but it has taken a good deal of time for that to happen. Baby loss certificates are now issued to parents who have lost a pregnancy, allowing them to formally recognise their loss.

It was a horrible time but we still had Sarah and Kelly to be mum and dad to, and we had to focus on that. I can't think of anything much more traumatic than losing two babies like that and, some months afterwards, Lyn was experiencing a lot of different symptoms which no one could initially explain. Apart from symptoms such as mood swings, which were an obvious link to losing the babies, she was very stressed. There was a good deal of depression, which was natural, given what had happened, and she sometimes seemed to have some difficulty walking.

This was a very challenging time for us both but particularly for Lyn, who was trying to come to terms with such a huge loss.

Many things were said, which she regretted; many things were thrown as well, but nothing caused any physical damage, apart from some dents in the furniture.

I suffered from that loss as well but, even now, the effect of miscarriage on a father is not recognised as much as it should be. Over the next couple of years, Lyn's symptoms increased; her moods changed very often and it was difficult to deal with, especially not knowing the cause and, therefore, no understanding of how to deal with it. She had also started experiencing some dizziness and more walking problems; nothing much to begin with, just there in the background. This was more than post-partum depression…

On reflection, I think that the GP should have put Lyn, or both of us, in touch with a therapist to talk it all through at regular sessions. This is certainly what would happen now but was not the case at that time.

Although there was clearly something going on with Lyn's health, throughout 1986 she wanted to get back to work and rejoined the Civil Service—at the Department of Employment in Milton Keynes—with the help of a childminder to look after Sarah and Kelly after school. She was there for a year or so, but it must be said that they were not her happiest times at work. She had a very difficult manager, who did not make her life any easier, to the point where, after much discussion between us, she initiated an internal complaint through her union. This resulted in the form of a disciplinary hearing that went against the manager, but it did not help Lyn. If anything, it made her worse, as she was constantly worrying about her inability to keep up with her work targets, with seemingly very little support from her colleagues or line managers.

It can be very difficult working in that kind of environment when you are not feeling yourself, for some unexplained reason, and with very little understanding about how this is affecting you. That kind of attitude from an employer and a manager was unacceptable then and it certainly would be now. If anyone feels they are not being treated fairly or not being listened to, they should report it to their employers, who are legally obliged to investigate and make changes to the working environment if necessary.

Lyn was effectively forced to leave as she was 'not performing' and life was made very difficult for her, a disgraceful decision on the part of a government department. While not an excuse, that is how it was at that time. She had to leave as the situation was doing her no good whatsoever.

Sarah was now seven and had been at school for a couple of years; Kelly was almost five and had only just started at the local infants school (first school now). It was quite a good school, but we had been talking to friends and neighbours who had children of varying school ages; there seemed to be a general feeling that the Milton Keynes education system was not good enough. We carefully considered our options and realised that we had built up a sizeable equity in our self-build house, so we started thinking seriously about what to do next.

We knew that Harrow's education system was good; it went into the melting pot and, in 1986, we decided to move back. We sold our house in Milton Keynes quite quickly, too quickly, in fact, to allow us to find somewhere straight away in Harrow Weald, where we used to live. We moved in, temporarily, with my dad, having stored all our worldly goods in the spare rooms at Lyn's grandad's flat in Belmont, Harrow Weald. We managed to move ourselves—and all those worldly goods—in a large Ford Transit box van and our car.

After a couple of months of searching, we found our ideal house in Harrow Weald; the first and middle schools were, conveniently and literally, at the end of our road, and we were only fifteen minutes' walk from the high school that Lyn had attended.

We had many happy times in that house, as Sarah and Kelly grew up, and we all made more friends.

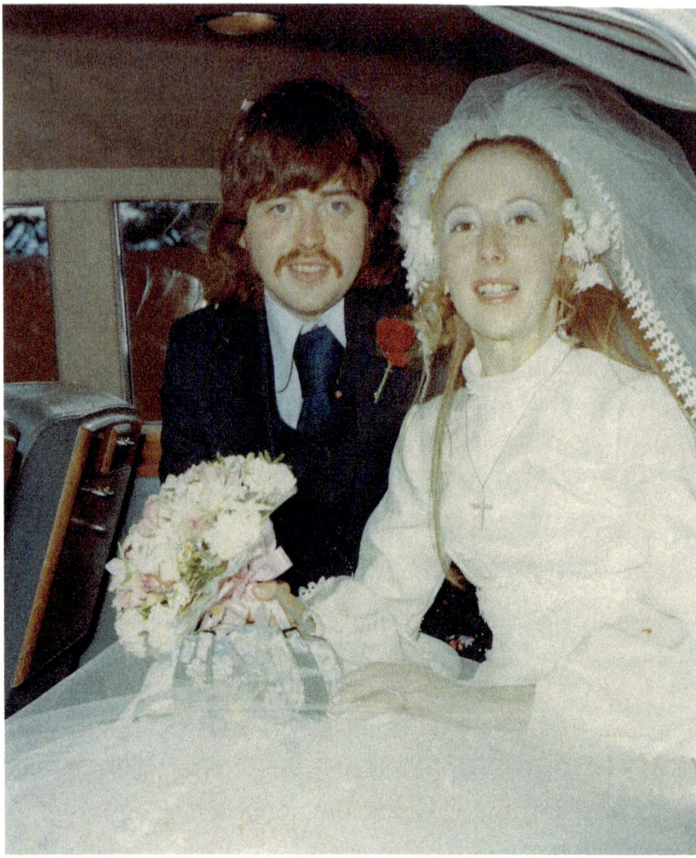

Our wedding day, 1974.

6 The MS diagnosis

There has been much anecdotal evidence from friends and people with MS, whom we met over the years, and from anecdotal evidence in publications, that MS of whatever type may have been triggered by a traumatic event in their lives. This could certainly have been the case with Lyn; losing the twins was certainly the most traumatic event in her life up to that point. There does not seem to be any medical evidence to prove this, but it does seem more than coincidental.

It was probably a year or two after losing the twins that we really started noticing some odd symptoms: Lyn's balance was becoming more affected, dizziness, more fatigue and some difficulty in walking, odd feelings in her hands that she just started to call 'buzzy'. To Lyn, that is what it was, a buzzing feeling, like a very low electrical current passing down her arms to her hands and fingers. She also had problems with her right leg, which seemed to drag occasionally.

In 1989, after several discussions with our GP about Lyn's symptoms, Lyn was referred to a consultant at the National Hospital for Nervous Diseases (now the National Hospital for Neurology and Neurosurgery) in Queen's Square in London, where she had an MRI scan. I have to say that the consultant who delivered the initial diagnosis, following the scan, was not the most sympathetic. He looked at his desk rather than at Lyn when he told us that it was MS. Lyn was shocked, to say the least, and there was little explanation, compassion, or anything else. I don't think either of us took in what was being said or the real impact; he simply said that Lyn should contact her GP again to discuss prescriptions and so on...

Whether it was a sign of the times or not, his manner was far from satisfactory. Lyn was clearly shocked by the diagnosis and all I could think of was getting her out of there and consoling her. We left the hospital in a daze; we had just been told, in the most basic way, that Lyn had MS, without much of an explanation or advice about what was going to happen in the future or what we could do to find out more.

We talked it through that evening; Lyn called the surgery in the morning and made an appointment for the following afternoon with our GP to discuss what was happening to her. At the end of the appointment, during which there was minimal discussion, he just handed her a leaflet and said, 'These people might be able to help.' It was an MS Society leaflet…

I can remember coming home from work that evening and being surprised to see one of Lyn's friends in the kitchen, with an arm protectively around Lyn's shoulders. Her friend stayed while Lyn explained what had happened at the GP's surgery. We did have another meeting with the GP, when there was a little more explanation and he suggested we contact the MS Society to get more information about the disease. He also prescribed some initial medication: Beta Interferon, which is used to dampen inflammation, and Baclofen, to relieve spasms, cramping and tightening of muscles, which Lyn found she could not tolerate as it made her dizzy; it also made her fatigue worse.

Everyone reacts differently to medications and you do not know until you have tried it if something will work for you, so Lyn would always try medications that were recommended.

The whole situation at that time was very difficult; Lyn had just been diagnosed with something that neither she nor I fully understood. We had two young daughters: Sarah, who was eleven at the time, and Kelly, who was only nine. How were we going to explain what was happening to Lyn if we, ourselves, did not know?

I suppose it is the same with anything; someone mentions a disease and you just register the name. Unless it happens to you, or someone close to you, there is rarely, if ever, a need to understand more—but now we had to. We had heard of it but did not understand what it really meant. There were many tears and that is to be expected something totally unexpected has hit you.

I needed to try to find out as much as I could, so I could do my best to understand what Lyn was going through, and what to expect, so that I would know how to help her. We contacted the MS Society, who were very good; the society arranged to send us a pack of advisory booklets that described the different types of MS and the different symptoms of each type, as well information on exercise, diet and so on—all aspects of the disease.

We read the leaflets, which were well produced and easy to read. Lyn was not an avid reader; she never enjoyed reading for pleasure, but she wanted to find out more and did try to take in what she could. She often said, and it was true, that the only time she ever read was to study, not for enjoyment, and now, with her fatigue symptoms getting noticeably worse, she found it difficult to concentrate and absorb what she was reading. I have always enjoyed reading and so I read as much as I could to try to understand what we were dealing with, what we could do about it, and what the future might hold. I had to fully understand it all, as much as I could, to be able to help Lyn to understand.

This was a very difficult time, as we did not know what might lay ahead; we could not hide things from the girls, and we had to talk to them in simple terms about MS. These are all difficult things to process when you are an adult, even more so as a child, and they found it hard, Sarah struggled more than Kelly at that time, as she was a little older and had more of an understanding of what was happening to her mum. At eleven years old, Sarah was going through her own changes; her hormones were going up and down, her periods had started, and her teenage years lay ahead.

There were times, shortly after Lyn was diagnosed, when both girls found it all very confusing and difficult to deal with. There was also some anger, probably due to their frustration in seeing what was happening to their mum and that there was nothing much that they could do about it.

Sarah reacted in a somewhat rebellious way, lashing out against what was happening. There were some issues with authority at school, and she was asked to leave the Girl Guides for the same reason. She still has an issue with authority figures...

As the girls moved into their early teens and then on to their later teenage years, Lyn and I could always talk to them about everything, with no holds barred and no embarrassment. It has carried on ever since. The girls have often said that some of their friends would never dream of talking about their periods and that kind of stuff to their dad. I do not know why; I have always tried to be open about everything. Why would you not? Also, at that age, children think that their parents are invincible, heroes even, and that they are going to be there forever, so when something like MS comes along, it upsets everything. From the outset, once we had talked things through in terms they could understand, Sarah and Kelly were incredibly supportive and protective of Lyn; they knew that life had changed and that they needed to step up.

They knew it was not a babying thing or a need to wrap her in cotton wool, it was just understanding that things had changed, that mum sometimes needed to rest, that she could not walk as far as she used to, and that sometimes she was very tired or a little upset. Both Lyn and I were, and always remained, very proud of how our girls dealt with everything at the time and over the years.

Shortly after Lyn's diagnosis, the MS Society also put us in touch with its Harrow branch, the local support group; it held regular monthly social meetings and we went to the next one. About twenty people attended; some were in wheelchairs, which was rather disconcerting, as the first thing you tend to think is, 'This is my future?' It is upsetting and daunting for someone who is newly diagnosed.

Lyn and I were always quite pragmatic about things; we would deal with them head on, so she put the wheelchair thing aside and simply talked to people.

Some people do not find it easy to talk and open up to their relatives and those closest to them; sometimes, they may find it easier talking to someone who is not so close to what is happening. That is where the local MS Society support groups can help, as there are other people who are going through the same thing and are they quite happy to talk about their MS. From what I learned of local MS Society branches, they are always welcoming and will try and put you at your ease. It is very important to talk to other people; if you do not, you bottle up everything, which is not good for your mental health.

At this same time, the early stages of Lyn's MS were showing many different symptoms. Lyn had also been suffering increasingly from premenstrual tension (PMT) and was starting to go through the initial stages of early menopause. Apart from the fact that her periods had started to become heavier, with intermittent bleeding as well, there were also several menopausal symptoms that were very similar to those of MS. Anxiety, mood swings, fatigue—it was very difficult and quite confusing for Lyn and me, trying to differentiate between the two things that were affecting her. Living with MS is one thing; living with MS and PMT and going through early menopause is something entirely different.

This was possibly the worst time of our lives as there was so much to try and deal with; it caused a good deal of tension between us. Understandably, this led to plenty of frustration on Lyn's part and on mine. She also became anxious and quite depressed about everything; as a result, her GP prescribed Sertraline, which she took for about six months. It helped, but only to the extent that it gradually decreased her anxiety; there were still the underlying issues to deal with.

Push came to shove when this had been going on for over a year. Lyn was suffering but I was fortunate to have private medical insurance through the company I worked for. Lyn got a referral to see a gynaecologist at the Clementine Churchill Hospital in Harrow in early 1994. As usual, I went with Lyn to the consultation, not just for support, but also to understand exactly what was going on. The gynaecologist recommended that Lyn have a hysterectomy—just the uterus, not a full pelvic clearance, which could have caused her even more long-term complications.

I had already booked a holiday in Cyprus, and I wanted to make sure that Lyn's operation was carried out well before then, so that she would have time to recuperate. Fortunately, I was able to contact the consultant; she understood the situation and very kindly fitted Lyn into her schedule. She performed the operation at exactly the right time, so Lyn had a lovely relaxing break in the sun to start her recovery.

During the year after Lyn's hysterectomy, we were able to fully focus on her MS and how it was affecting her. Now we needed to try to ascertain exactly what type of MS she had and what the future would be like. With the medical insurance, I was able to get a consultation.

In 1995 she was admitted to the National Hospital for Nervous Diseases (now the National Hospital for Neurology and Neurosurgery) in Queen Square, London, for tests, including an MRI scan and a lumbar puncture. To confirm a primary progressive MS diagnosis, an MRI scan must show two or more lesions appearing in different parts of the brain or spinal cord at different times. A lumbar puncture must also show signs of MS (antibodies) in the fluid around the spinal cord. Lyn was diagnosed with primary progressive MS.

At the time, she was under the care of Professor Alan Thompson, who is still at the hospital. He had become a leading light into MS research and is now the Dean of the Faculty of Brain Sciences at University College Hospital, London. In 2021 he received the Charcot Award, which is viewed by the MS community as the ultimate accolade for a lifetime's work into the research and treatment of this disease.

Leaving the hospital, Lyn and I were both in a daze. While we now knew exactly what Lyn had, what did this new diagnosis mean for Lyn's future? We needed to find out more. Her consultant, from then on, was Dr Raj Kapoor, a good man who was also involved in MS research. He had a wonderful way with patients, putting them at their ease, while calmly discussing their case and including their husband or partner in that discussion. Nothing was ever rushed; he would always talk everything through with you. Lyn saw him or one of his colleagues frequently for the next fifteen years. Dr Kapoor has now retired but he was a professor at the National Hospital for Neurology and Neurosurgery in London until 2018 and by then, I would think, even more respected than when we knew him.

It was very important for me to be part of the discussion about Lyn's MS with whoever we consulted, as her short-term memory was not that great. It had definitely become worse over time—a side effect of MS? Yes, although, at the time, I could not be sure of that. It was essential for me to understand what was being discussed or happening so that

I could help Lyn to understand, as she would sometimes be a little confused, or forget to tell the consultant about aspects of her condition or symptoms, which might be of use to them in her continuing treatment.

Some people with MS find it hard to find the right words, to concentrate or to recall things that might be important for the consultant to know, to enable them to come to the right conclusion. I never had any objections from doctors or consultants about my being part of the consultation process; I think they feel it is better for the wider family understanding of a condition, as this can only help the patient. If you do go for a consultation, never worry about taking your spouse or a close friend; anything that can help you understand what is being discussed can only be good.

7 Life with MS, the early years

With Lyn's hysterectomy now out of the way, and with her diagnosis of primary progressive MS, we could concentrate on how she could deal with her MS, from day to day. We now knew exactly what primary progressive MS was, and we knew what the symptoms were, and which of them would become progressively worse over the years.

There were, understandably, many things that we had to adjust to in the first few years as Lyn's MS progressed. She had now also been diagnosed with an under-active thyroid. This was another blow; when we investigated, there were again some symptoms very similar to MS: fatigue, muscle aches and pains, cognitive and physical impairments and depression. Here we would go again, trying to differentiate between symptoms. Thankfully, Levothyroxine, the medication that she was prescribed, controlled many of the symptoms, although it was cumulative and took about six weeks to take effect.

As we had always shared domestic tasks, there was a transition over time, with me gradually taking on more of the tasks that Lyn was finding difficult. We take for granted the simple things of everyday life until MS starts to develop.

Vacuuming

With Lyn's balance difficulties, this was becoming impossible; the idea of her standing up, concentrating on staying upright and using the vacuum cleaner hose and attachments, while trying to remember where the electric lead was and not tripping over it, was an accident waiting to happen.

Cleaning bathrooms

It was much the same problem; when Lyn was bending over and cleaning the bath and toilet, she always experienced a sense of vertigo. She would feel unbalanced, probably try to stand up too quickly, feel a bit dizzy, and possibly fall over.

Cooking

We had always shared the cooking. When I was working full time in London, Lyn would sometimes cook for the girls before I got home, or I would prepare something the night before so she could just heat it up. Most of the time, we all managed to eat together, which was important for us.

So generally, there was a good deal of preparation the night before and some heating up the following day; if the weather was warm, salads were always a good standby. For their future benefit and to help us, we had always taught Sarah and Kelly to help with preparation and cooking, and they were always willing to do this. They have both become very good cooks over the years.

Before Lyn's MS developed, she always like to cook traditional meals, such as roasts and casseroles, while I prepared mainly Indian, Chinese and other types of dishes.

As time progressed it became all too clear that, with Lyn's balance and dexterity issues, the idea of her working in a kitchen with sharp knives, moving a pan of boiling hot water or pasta or taking something hot out of the oven, for example, was not a good idea.

We worked out a compromise; Lyn would help with the prep work, such as cutting up veggies, and some of the cooking, as long as it did not involve carrying anything hot. It is incredibly important for anyone with any type of MS to still feel part of whatever is happening so, although Lyn realised that she could not do much in the kitchen, she remained involved by deciding what to have for dinner that day and helping with the preparation. In Harrow Weald, we had a kitchen breakfast bar, where she used to sit to do any prepping; she could look out onto the garden from there as well, which always gave her pleasure. We also bought a perching stool, which meant that, when it was safe enough, she could sit in front of the hob, as well as the worktop, at a slightly raised level to do some cooking.

Lyn had wanted to start working again and, in 1988, she got a job within the Civil Service at the Department of Work and Pensions (DWP) in Harrow. Unfortunately, the manager she had suffered under in Milton Keynes was now working there! Not a happy start but the manager left soon after she joined and Lyn stuck with the job for a few years. She liked working; Lyn wanted to feel that she was doing something positive with her life and contributing something to our household funds.

As a people person, generally, Lyn liked the people she worked with and liked meeting people, but it became obvious that her MS had deteriorated to the extent that it was impacting on her ability to work. Her walking and balance were now compromised and she increasingly used a walking stick; the demands of the job, and the stress involved in dealing with members of the public who were, shall we say, not the nicest to deal with on certain occasions, were all beginning to take their toll. In fact, sometimes it was positively dangerous…thankfully, the DWP decided to install screens at the public counters, as some claimants had jumped over the counter, aggrieved at being told that they were not entitled to a payment.

In 1993, Lyn decided to cut her hours but, even working part time, her fatigue was becoming more of an issue, making it difficult for her to fulfil her job description and function. We had known, for some time, through the local MS Society branch, that there was plenty of help and advice for people with different disabilities, not just MS, about working or not working and claiming benefits. At that time, there was a general feeling among most people of our age that you should work if you could and not be reliant upon the benefits system. The flipside is that you have worked and contributed to society all of your working life up to that time, so now that you need help why should you not apply for it?

Simple? Absolutely not. The benefits system, at that time, for people with disabilities, was a nightmare and difficult to understand—even for Lyn, who had worked within the system for years. It was a minefield. The bottom line then was, and probably still is now, that no-one in the benefits system will tell you what you are entitled to, unless you ask specific questions. No information was volunteered on what might be available—unless you actually applied. Similarly, the forms were, and probably still are, lengthy and difficult for anyone to understand, let alone someone with a disability that affects their mental capacity and memory. I suspect that many people over the years have probably thought about making a claim for some kind of benefit to suit their own personal circumstances…but have been put off by the bureaucracy involved in completing the forms, especially as they are just handed over, with no advice or help on how to complete them.

We were put in contact with a wonderful lady called Gladys Janes, who was working for the Harrow Association of Disabled People. This was a wonderful organisation, which still exists today. Gladys Janes, became a trustee, was awarded an MBE for services to the community, and has now retired. The association acted as a go-between for people with any kind of disability and social and council services, providing advice and support, mentally and practically, and essential help in completing benefit application forms. We made an appointment and had a couple of sessions with Gladys, which she then followed up.

The bottom line was that Lyn could apply for a couple of different benefits that, combined with her medical early retirement payments from the Civil Service, would enable her to take medical retirement and receive almost the same amount of money each month that she had received as a salary with the DWP. It was a no-brainer; Lyn handed in her notice and took early medical retirement in 1996. With Gladys's help, we completed the forms and, after a few months, the benefits started to be paid, backdated to the time of the claim.

What a difference that made. Lyn was no longer stressed by having to go to work; she was a more relaxed and, although she missed working with people and her friends, it was more important to be what she wanted to be, and do what she wanted to do, within her limitations. It opened up a whole new world for her.

One door closes and another one opens was a saying that summed up Lyn's approach to life. Always look for ways in which you can improve your circumstances and never let your disability define you.

In the same year, 1996, my dad passed away; he had had an operation in 1991 for stomach cancer and, after the five years they had predicted, he succumbed again—another sad time for our family.

Thank goodness for the help we received in obtaining benefit support. If you need any help with the benefits system or making a claim, I would urge you to make contact with either the MS Society or Citizens Advice, or any disability advice organisation. There is no point in trying to do this on your own and banging your head against the wall; talk to people who know the system and can help. It could make a massive and positive difference to your life and wellbeing.

Another valuable thing that Lyn did was to give a talk, followed by a question and answer session, to trainee doctors at our local GP practice about MS from an 'expert patient' point of view. The surgery knew of our involvement with the local MS support group and was keen to help local people with MS. That initial talk was very well received, and, over the years, the practice asked Lyn back every couple of months.

In 1998, Lyn's balance issues once caused a serious problem. She was downstairs, and Sarah and I were upstairs when we heard a loud moan, followed by a thump. We rushed downstairs to find Lyn on the dining room floor with a pool of blood spreading around her head. While Sarah called 999, I put some clean towels around Lyn's head; we could not see where the wound was as there was so much blood.

As it was a head injury, the operator wanted me to keep talking to Lyn, asking her questions to make sure she kept awake and that she was still cognisant. The ambulance soon arrived and, after some initial checks, the paramedics slid a solid stretcher under her and used a collar to support her head for transport. I followed the ambulance to the hospital, illegally going through the red lights directly behind them. I should not have done so but, understandably, I was not really bothered about the consequences.

At about midnight, we were in an A&E side room at Northwick Park Hospital; Lyn had been stabilised and the bleeding had stopped. The consultant could see that the actual wound was on the top of her forehead and, thankfully, under the hairline above her left eye. Once she had been cleaned up, a large flap of skin was visible. The consultant said that it was a large wound, which, because of its position, would need careful stitching—so she would be doing it herself. However, they were short of staff and I would have to help her! So, following her instructions, I scrubbed my hands, put on a blue gown, and there we were: the consultant was working away at the business end, shaving Lyn's hair, injecting anaesthetic around the wound and squirting it under the flap of skin that I was holding up out of the way, with a pair of stainless-steel forceps.

Lyn, who was fully awake, asked if everything was all

right.

'Well, it all looks OK from here,' said the consultant. 'What do you think?' she said, looking at me. There are probably few men who can say that they have seen their wife's skull.

'It's a sort of pinky-grey colour,' was all I could say.

Eighteen stitches later, all was well, and we went home. By the time we arrived, Sarah, Kelly, and her boyfriend, Keith, had worked hard and completely cleaned all evidence of blood from the carpet.

The next morning Lyn was able to explain that she had lost her balance and fallen back, onto the door frame, then bounced forward. As she fell, she had tried to scalp herself on the metal keep tab on the opposite frame. She wore bandanas made from scarves for some months, until her hair had grown back; it was a very attractive look. Luckily, she had always liked and bought scarves, so she had quite a collection.

I was now a senior surveyor / architectural designer with the same company in London; they were absolutely brilliant and made plenty of allowances. I adjusted my hours so that I could go in early, around 8.00am, and leave promptly at 5.00pm—to make sure that I got home as soon as possible. I always managed to keep up with my work, even if I had to work at home in the evenings; I had been with the company for twenty years and many of my colleagues had come to know Lyn very well.

In 1995, I had had an accident that caused a bad dislocation of the navicular bone in my right foot but, after a couple of operations, I was able to get back to normal life, with the aid of a walking stick, when necessary.

However, I had to give up working in London in 1999, as I could no longer carry out site inspections, up ladders and scaffolding. I decided to start my own business, working from home and concentrating on the design stages of the projects in which I was involved.

In a way, this made it easier for us to manage our lives and made perfect sense, as I could be there on hand to help Lyn during the day. This was becoming necessary as her MS symptoms were becoming worse, and I was able to carry on doing the work that I loved.

Many people I have spoken to over the years said that they would have found it difficult being under the same roof with their spouse for that amount of time. We were never together 24/7, as we both had our own interests to occupy our time; I would be working in one room, while Lyn and her computer were in another room, and sometimes one or other of us would be busy away from the house or meeting people about work or MS-related issues or seeing friends. We were very lucky to have achieved a work-life balance that suited us both. I was able to do what I wanted workwise and be there to help Lyn whenever she needed it, whether with everyday activities, personal care, or helping her get ready for the day or bedtime.

I did the vacuuming and cleaning at the weekends while I was working but, after considering how best to deal with this, we decided it was far better to find someone to help. We hired a local lady, who came in every week to tackle the cleaning. Maureen was a kind soul who did not have a bad bone in her body and was very helpful. She did three hours twice a week but could talk for England—and she used to get quite a few words wrong in any conversation! On one occasion, I was working in the office downstairs and had just spent a day writing a specification. Maureen stuck her head round the door and started talking without warning, just as I was about to press 'save'. What did I press? 'Don't save.' Aaaaaargh! Another time, she kept trying to tell me about an operation she was due to have but she could not remember what it was… Eventually, she shouted from the top of the stairs, 'I remember now, I've got a cartridge in my knee!'

When caring for someone, you need to be well yourself to be able to do it effectively.

In 2008, I had been having aches and pains and had swollen joints in my hands, knees and elbows. My knuckles were also very swollen and painful. This went on for some months and, despite several visits to the GP, there was little success in finding out what was wrong. All I knew was that it severely limited everything I did or wanted to do. My hands were so badly affected that I could not move them easily; I could not draw, paint or play the guitar and, more important, it affected my ability to help Lyn.

After leaving the firm I had worked for in London, I continued paying for private medical cover. I asked my GP for a referral to see a consultant and was referred to a rheumatologist. After an initial consultation, the rheumatologist arranged for me to have CT scans and blood tests. At the follow-up appointment some weeks later, he told me that I had rheumatoid arthritis, an autoimmune disease, in which the body's immune system attacks itself.

The immune system helps to defend our body from infections. But, in rheumatoid arthritis, the immune system sends antibodies to the lining of the joints by mistake. The antibodies then attack the tissues surrounding the joint. This causes the thin layer of cells (synovium) covering the joints to become sore and inflamed. Inflammation also causes chemicals to be released. These chemicals thicken the synovium and damage the joints.

The consultant prescribed Methotrexate, a chemotherapy drug, which—in lower doses—helps to alleviate the rheumatoid arthritis symptoms. After some months, I began to get the movement back in my joints and the pain decreased. It was not completely back to normal but at least I could use my hands more easily; the swelling in my knees and elbows reduced considerably and, over the next twelve years, my condition improved.

8 The MS Society

The MS Society proved to be an invaluable source of information for us in the first few months after Lyn's diagnosis and remained so. The society has raised its profile over the years and today most people have at least heard of it and the work it does.

As I have said, until something happens to you there is no real need to find out more; once it does happen, you need to find out everything possible to try to understand what you are dealing with, what the symptoms are, how they will affect you, whether everyone feels the same, will it get worse, how soon, is it terminal? All these thoughts go through your mind, as someone with MS and as a husband, wife, partner, girlfriend or boyfriend.

The MS Society produces helpful information in booklets, covering every aspect of MS: the different types, how the symptoms differ, diet, nutrition, treatments and therapies, and pain management, for example. The list is too long to include here; suffice it to say it covers as much as is known about MS. This is an extract from the society's website:

> Here to help you manage your MS
> We want to:
>
> > Support you to build on your understanding of your MS and share your knowledge with other people
> > Support you to make informed choices about your

care and treatment, including disease modifying therapies (DMTs)
Suggest ways to improve your emotional wellbeing and build resilience, so you can deal with whatever life with MS throws at you

Give you space to connect with our community, a network of people who know MS and can support you through your journey

Lessen the financial impact of MS by helping you find ways to stay in work, go back to work or claim benefits to help you live a more independent life
help you find ways to be physically active that fit in with your life.

Our service charter
Planning our services together:
We value your experience and knowledge and always want to hear your views

We'll regularly find ways to talk to you about how we can improve, to make sure our services are meeting your needs. You can contact us anytime, by email phone or social media to share your thoughts and feedback.

We want to make sure our services are open to everyone who needs them. We'll work with you to understand how best we can do this

Making our services work for everyone:
We'll follow best practice to deliver quality services that make a real difference to people's lives

We'll treat you with courtesy, fairness and respect

We won't judge you, or treat one person more favourably than another

We'll communicate with you the way you tell us works best for you keeping your personal data safe

We take our commitment to you very seriously and will take every step to guard your personal information

We'll never sell or swap your personal details with another organisation, and will only share your data when you have given us permission to do so

We'll only ever contact you through channels you are happy for us to use

If you don't want to hear from us, then you just need to tell us over the phone or by email

Always here to listen:

We want you to tell us when we get it right or wrong so we can continue to improve

We'll always be friendly and open when you get in

touch

We'll get back to you in good time and let you know what we're going to do with what you told us

We'll use your feedback to help shape and develop our services

Got something to tell us?

Contact the MS Society Supporter care team

You can talk to or email the MS Society about anything that concerns you and it will point you in the right direction. I would strongly urge anyone who is either newly diagnosed or a carer for someone in that position to contact the MS Society, it could help to change your lives. There are booklets and factsheets about all aspects of MS; you can order hard copies by telephone or online or download and print hard copies.

9 Helping with the local branch of the MS Society

Once we had started to go to the MS Society branch's monthly social meetings, we realised just how many local people were affected by MS in varying degrees. There were probably thirty to forty people who attended the meetings and there were also those who were housebound. You begin to wonder…if this is the case locally, how many people are affected across the UK or the world?

The local branch had been going for several years by then; there was a chairman, a treasurer, a secretary, and volunteers who helped in various ways. They used to meet at a building owned by Harrow Council; on weekdays, it acted as a day centre for people with various special needs, and the local MS branch had the use of it all day on Saturdays once a month.

Over the next few months, we learned that some of the volunteers were widows, widowers or simply friends of members who had MS (or had passed away over the years) and they wanted to carry on helping others, which was a wonderful thing to do. Initially, it was probably not the kind of social gathering you would want to go to out of choice but you always meet people and make friends, sometimes for life—just like the school playground.

There were many members of that local branch who had relapsing remitting MS; there were some who had primary progressive MS like Lyn, and there were others who were wheelchair bound or housebound and had secondary progressive MS. Lyn had a way with people, even on first acquaintance. She loved a chat over a cup of tea and some cake; she felt part of the group straight away engendering a need in her to help others. Lyn soon made friends with everyone in that group and so did I. The common bond was, of course, MS and what a horrible disease it is, whichever type you have. Lyn's initial chats with everybody were based around that; for example, what type did they have, how it affected them, their symptoms, what their GP was like, who was their consultant and what were they like?

We got to know many people over the years when we were involved with the local branch; not all had MS, some were helpers or committee members from other branches and some have remained friends to this day. As Lyn was still able to walk without a stick sometimes, in the early to mid-1990s, we would help at the socials, serving tea, sandwiches and the ever-present cakes. There was much laughter at those meetings, a sense of 'Just get on with your life while you can and don't let the bastards get you down.' Lyn's attitude was always do what you can, when you can, for as long as you can; we shared a similar attitude and outlook on life.

Every year, all the branch members were invited to a large house in Northwood Hills, owned by a doctor friend of the branch treasurer. It was a fine house in its own grounds, with plenty of room for members' children to run around. It also had a swimming pool, which was well used at those functions. The first time we went, we did the normal parental thing, warning the girls—they were about fourteen and twelve—to be on their best behaviour and mind their Ps and Qs.

The girls were quite happy to help serve refreshments to members who were wheelchair bound, one of whom was Clive. He was an interesting character, quite severely disabled, but he never seemed to let it affect him. Clive was also known to smoke the odd joint, as he was convinced it was helping—nothing wrong with that.

Sarah asked Clive what he wanted to drink.

'Oh, I'll have a beer, please.'

She brought the beer, poured it into the glass and handed it to him.

'Thanks.'

As he took the glass, his hand shook uncontrollably and the beer spilled down his shirt front and onto his trousers.

'Oh, fuck!' he said loudly.

The girls looked at me in horror, rarely having heard the word, and certainly not in public from an adult. So much for best behaviour.

We went for several years, until the doctor's ill health brought these annual events to an end.

On another occasion, Clive attended one of the branch's guest speaker sessions, given this time by Dr Raj Kapoor, who was giving a talk on the possible benefits of cannabis or cannabinoids on MS.

'So, has anyone here ever tried cannabis?' he asked.

A voice from the back said, 'Oh yeah man, I smoke it all the time.' Predictably, it was Clive.

When Lyn and I helped with the local branch, we were involved in different and similar roles. Lyn was now keen to help others in the MS community; she was already a member of the local branch committee and volunteered to take over producing the monthly newsletter. She began with what had been done before but could see that there was room for improvement. She started by looking at newsletters from other local branches and talking to their editors and the MS Society. The result was a very impressive newsletter, which was informative about different aspects of MS, new research, and carried articles from members and other contributors. In short, it was brilliant and very well received; it was circulated to members, the local GP practice, which was supportive, and the MS Society and other branches where she had developed contacts.

As Lyn was now free from work-related stress, she felt she had the time to try to do more to help other members, so she became involved with the branch's welfare activities. She built up a remarkable network of people, either with MS or with links to it and would often spend a few hours each morning, talking to people on the telephone or emailing them, or researching something on the internet. Inevitably, this would sometimes take its toll and she would not feel like doing much for the rest of the day—but that is the nature of MS. You try to pace yourself and it might work, then life gets in the way; something else comes up that you've got to deal with and you are back to square one. You might be too tired to go back to the thing you were doing in the first place; nevertheless life goes on, day by day.

If you get a chance to help in any way at a local support branch, I recommend that you do so. I am sure they would welcome you with open arms, as there are far more people needing various types of help than volunteers willing and able to help.

As I mentioned, one thing that has never ceased to

amaze me is the amount of bureaucracy that someone has to fight through to get anywhere with the benefits system. I lost count of the number of times I had to help members fill out forms; luckily, we had the likes of Gladys Janes and, if she could not help, Citizens Advice was always on hand. Call me a cynic, but it always seemed to me that the forms were deliberately designed to catch people out. There could be four or five ten to twenty-page sections in most application forms for disability benefits; each section was worded differently and with a different slant—but largely about the same thing—to all appearances as if they were trying to trip you…Or was it simply that there was no consideration of, or input from, the end user? The forms were simply not fit for purpose. I have not had to deal with things like this for some years but I suspect they are still written in the same way.

There was a good deal to do, helping the local branch, but not many people available to help. I drove the branch bus for about five years; it was quite old but had a low mileage and had been given to the branch some years before. I had to follow the Public Service Vehicle Health and Safety guidelines and we had to spend a fair amount of money on special wheelchair restraints that kept the chairs safely bolted to the floor during trips. We used it for several years as it supplemented the Harrow Council monthly bus allocation, which the branch was entitled to. I used to drive members to monthly meetings, social events at other branches, trips and to respite care homes. The council provided this transport for member groups and organisations. The service provided accessible minibuses (up to sixteen passenger seats) for local and national journeys, such as shopping, meetings, lunch clubs, or local visits, summer camps, and day trips, including visits to the coast.

Group transport was open to all voluntary, community, statutory and other not-for-profit organisations in the London Borough of Harrow and its environs. Providing buses for people with disabilities was an essential lifeline for many in Harrow; for example, to help disabled people access various support services on weekdays. On Saturdays, the council also offered a regular monthly service to local groups that needed help with transport, which enabled our members to get to the monthly meetings. As far as I know, Harrow still provides this service and it would be worth checking with your local council to see if it offers something similar.

These trips might often be the only way that some members without any family support could get out of their homes and meet other people. I think we sometimes take our ease of access to everything we need and want for granted; it is only when you see how some people have to manage their lives that you realise how lucky you are.

Eventually we had to give up the bus, as it was becoming uneconomical to run when setting the costs of fuel, maintenance and insurance against the use and benefit. It was better for us to pay the council for an additional bus when it was needed.

As well as producing the newsletter, Lyn was also one of four committee members helping with welfare; they worked in pairs for safety reasons. This was quite an involved role, as it meant visiting branch members in their homes with another committee member, assessing what members' needs were and what help they needed. Lyn and her colleagues would then liaise with the committee, the MS Society and social services to put things in place. This sometimes meant liaising with care services, for example, or helping people obtain grants for equipment in their homes, either from local branch funds or from the MS Society. Lyn carried out this role for about five years and I would sometimes get involved, if she needed help. If there was one thing that worried me about Lyn dealing with these welfare issues, it was the amount of time it could take and the effect this was having on her and her symptoms.

The chairman at the time was eighty and he had been in the role for several years; understandably, he had been trying to get someone else to do the job for some time so, at one of the AGMs, I put myself forward. It was a role I enjoyed, helping to co-ordinate the other committee members and their activities, and trying to ensure that no-one was overloaded in their individual roles, including liaising with other branches and the national centre, and going to meetings. Unfortunately, it also had its downside as it was taking up to two days in time every week, while I was working almost full time and helping care for Lyn. It was very time consuming but I carried out this role for five years.

The MS Society held a national AGM, which Lyn and I attended for several years, representing the Harrow branch. This was a two-day event; we would go to the venue on the Friday, to avoid rushing around on the Saturday, before the AGM started. As well as the AGM, a speaker would give a talk on an aspect of MS and research updates, and there was the opportunity to catch up and network with other branches and talk to national centre staff about issues that affected the local branch. We used to put together an AGM précis for the committee and members, so that they could be kept up to date with what was happening.

One year the hotel provided a large number of accessible portaloos near a side entrance and the room we had for the AGM. I had seen *Dr Who* actor, Tom Baker, in the hotel so I could not resist going to reception and leaving a message that his new Tardis was waiting for him at the side entrance…

Getting involved in a local MS branch can be very rewarding. Just be wary of taking on too much. One of the most difficult, but most important, things you have to learn when volunteering is when to say no, otherwise you will be unable to carry out your role properly and you will get stressed. This is something you do not want as you are trying to help people with MS deal with their own stressful situations.

At the end of our time helping with the local branch, Lyn and I received the Mayor of Harrow's Award for Services to the Community. This recognised the contribution we had both made by helping with the Harrow branch of the MS Society. By this time, Lyn had been helping with the branch in various roles, for fifteen years, even with her disabilities.

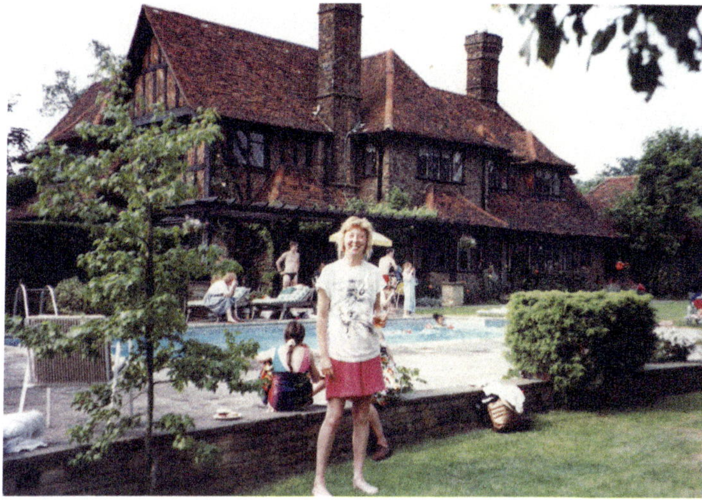

MS branch annual garden party, 1992.

10 Employment problems and disability

I have already mentioned Lyn's early problems with employment and MS, but she was far from alone. Several local branch members had experienced something similar.

In the late 1990s, one member, who had primary progressive MS, was still working as an electrical quantity surveyor for a large electrical contractor; he was in his mid-thirties and married, with two young children. He loved his job but was finding it increasingly difficult to get to work. Public transport was out of the question; he could still drive, but not confidently, nor for any distance, so he asked his company for help. It was patently obvious that they no longer wanted him to work for them, as they saw him as a liability, so they moved him to another job, which meant more travel. I think they offered to pay towards his taxi journeys, but the situation became untenable. Essentially, he was hounded out of his job. He received some compensation from an employment tribunal but it probably did not cover much.

This was not the only time that I came into contact with someone who had employment difficulties. The way employment law and the Disability Discrimination Act (DDA) have developed since their inception means that an employer must make allowances for an employee with a disability, ensure that they have easy access into their workplace, use of toilet facilities and so on, to make their working environment as comfortable to work in as it is for their colleagues.

With something like MS, the last thing you need is any additional stress in your life; this leads to your symptoms becoming worse, which then affects your performance at work; you worry more—because you feel you are not doing your job properly—which leads back to stress. It is a vicious circle. Employers must also consider 'reasonable' adjustments to a person's work role, namely training in another similar or even different role that suits you better.

The MS Society produces a booklet entitled *MS in the workplace: an employer's guide*. Here is an extract from the MS Society website:

> This booklet provides information for employers on employees affected by MS. It also has helpful information for health and social care professionals who work with people affected by MS.
>
> Download our MS in the workplace employer's guide for information about:
>
> What is MS
> MS and the law
> Working
> Everybody's rights and responsibilities
> How to support an employee with MS and 'reasonable adjustments'
> Practical tools and sources of support to help manage the impact of MS.
> It also has helpful information for health and social care professionals who work with people affected by MS.
> This booklet is available for you to download and print or you can order copies from our online shop. You can also

explore our webpages for more about MS in the workplace.

The Disability Discrimination Act, (DDA) and Employment Law covers this and provides protection for anyone with any kind of disability who feels aggrieved.

My job, at the time, involved a good deal of DDA work, namely surveys to ensure that buildings complied with the legislation to make the building, and access into and around it, easily accessible for anyone with a disability. This is not only for people with a mobility impairment, but also for anyone who is partially sighted or hearing impaired, for example. It covers not only building access but everything in the building, including lifts, fully accessible toilets, push button operated automatic doors, and manifestation to glass screens to help partially sighted people, all designed to enable anyone with any disability to negotiate their way into and around a building. Every owner of a building or premises used for their business has to ensure that, if they do not comply with DDA legislation and Part M of the Building Regulations, they must put a plan in place to make those necessary changes in a reasonable time.

Until DDA legislation came into effect, implementing this type of plan was purely voluntary but many large organisations had already started to do so. There were always businesses that did not want to comply, hence the need for legislation.

I heard something quite recently which was very worrying. A friend of mine attended a physio appointment at a local hospital; the doors into the unit from the corridor are heavy fire doors, but are not operated by an electric push button release. So she had to try and push them open and then had to bang on the door to attract attention. You would think that someone would have thought this one through and rectified it, before it became a problem in an environment where disabled access would be paramount.

DDA legislation covers not only a disabled person's right of access to a building but also that person's rights as an individual. The MS Society produces a booklet entitled *MS and your rights*. This is an extract from the MS Society website:

> If you have MS, the Equality Act or the Disability Discrimination Act can protect you against disability discrimination in education, work and services.
>
> These laws can make sure things are accessible for you and that you get reasonable adjustments and support from employers, colleges, venues and people who give you a service.
>
> Under the Equality Act you are also protected from discrimination if you are connected with someone who has a disability, like a family member or friend. And it can protect you if you've complained about discrimination or supported someone else's claim.
>
> The Equality Act applies in **England, Wales** and **Scotland**. In **Northern Ireland**, the Disability Discrimination Act applies.
>
> Is everyone with MS protected by the Equality Act? Yes. Some conditions like cancer, HIV and MS are automatically seen as disabilities under the Equality Act.
>
> There's no longer a national register of disabled people, so you don't need to register anywhere officially. But many local authorities do provide

help and support for disabled people, so it's worth contacting your local authority to find out how they can help you.

What counts as discrimination?

Discrimination is where you are treated unfairly and are put at a disadvantage when compared with people who aren't disabled.

You can be discriminated against:

Directly - if you are treated less well than others because you have MS. For example, if you are disciplined because you need to take more time off work than your colleagues to attend medical appointments

Indirectly – if your employer, college, venue or organisation has rules or arrangements in place which put you at an unfair disadvantage as a disabled person

If you are being harassed

If you are being victimised because you've complained about how you or someone else has been treated

What does the Equality Act cover?

Under the Act, disabled people should be treated equally. Protection from discrimination applies in many situations. These include buying or renting property, education, employment, goods, services, facilities and transport. It also covers things known as 'public functions', such as policing, planning applications with your local authority or receiving welfare benefits

You can't use the Act against an individual, like a neighbour who harasses you. Though you may be able to report it as a hate crime.

The Equality Act does cover harassment by an individual at a place where you work. If you think you've been unfairly discriminated against you can:

Complain directly to the person or organisation

Use someone else to help you sort it out - for example your union representative

Make a claim in a court or tribunal.

If you are in a position at work whereby your employer and their Human Resources department are not helping you with any difficulties you have, you are entitled to either speak to your union, if that is applicable or consult with Citizens Advice.

If neither your employer nor their human resources department are helping you with any difficulties you may have, it would be worth obtaining these booklets for your employer to ensure that they are aware of their legal responsibilities. You are also entitled to speak to your union representative, if applicable or to Citizens Advice.

11 Music, gigs and theatre

'If music be the food of love, play on…'
Twelfth Night, William Shakespeare

Lyn and I loved music; there was always a radio or CD playing music in the background during the day. She loved many kinds of music, which goes back to playing our records in those early days after we got together. Lyn was a romantic at heart and I suppose I am also a sucker for a good love song.

I went to so many gigs with my friends and then with Lyn, until we settled down to start a family, when much of what you would like to do goes on hold as life takes over. At some of the gigs, there were major names, such as Led Zeppelin. I had first seen them in 1969 at the Royal Albert Hall, one of their first major UK gigs and I took Lyn to see them at Wembley Arena, a year or so after we met, where she fell for the other man in her life—Robert Plant. We saw Robert at a gig with his band, Strange Sensation, at Somerset House in London in 2006 and I have seen him since.

As the girls grew up, they listened to the music we loved, anything from soul, Motown and R&B, to blues and melodic rock, some heavy rock, cool jazz and light classical music; all very eclectic. When the girls were in their teens, we took them to some small gigs in and around London, and some fairly major gigs too, at the old Wembley Stadium and Wembley Arena to see Toto,

Tina Turner, Bryan Adams, U2, Sheryl Crow and Rolling Stones among others. At the Tina Turner gig, Lyn and the girls were looking at her saxophone player on the big screen, who was bare chested; all his muscles were in the right place and, with his oiled skin and flowing hair, he looked like a rock god on the big screen. They were all drooling…

The great thing about these big gigs was that the disabled access arrangements were always very good; for example, clear access from car parking and entry onwards, seating in an area where you had a great view of the stage, and easy access to toilet facilities. This has improved so much since the DDA came into force, although there were quite a few venues that had already started doing much more voluntarily to improve access.

We continued to go to various gigs over the years: in 2004, memorable ones for Lyn, were Lionel Richie at Wembley Arena and Whitesnake at Hammersmith Apollo, two of her favourites.

Around 1997 I had also joined a band myself; like most other guys I knew at the time, I had dabbled with the guitar in my teens. I had bought an acoustic guitar a few years earlier and had been playing again. Now, with a chance to join a band at work for an organised party, I could get back to doing it again, could afford a decent guitar and amp, and had the time to practise. We stayed as a band, doing the pubs for a few years and even the odd corporate event, and used to meet regularly to rehearse, even if we were not gigging.

In the late 1990s, Lyn's MS was still fairly stable and I knew it was safe to leave her while I went to band 'reschmersals' as we called them, and she supported me in that. The rehearsal studio was only half an hour from home and she could always call her brother, Neil, or her friend, Val, if she needed any help. The other guys in the band knew about Lyn's MS and they and their partners were very understanding and supportive of her.

We even hired a recording studio and engineer in Berkshire one Sunday and recorded a three track CD as a demo; it was great fun and one of the best Sundays I can remember.

In 1996, our eldest daughter, Sarah, was at college doing her A-levels; we had played at a pub in St Albans quite a few times and even won a battle of the bands contest there. In fact, there were few bands in the contest but that was not the point: we won it. Sarah came along to the final with some of her friends and one of them, Keith, met Kelly, our younger daughter, that night. The rest is history, as they have been together ever since.

Sarah met her future husband, Steve, in 1999 on a holiday with some girlfriends; one day, they were on the beach and she was bored, just sitting around. Sarah spotted a group of lads playing footie, approached Steve, with one of her friends, and said, 'Can we play with you?' And that was the beginning of another history...

Lyn did not always feel up to going to local gigs so, knowing she was fine at home, with support if needed—and we never went far away—I took Sarah and Kelly to few gigs on their own which they enjoyed.

In the early 2000s, we were members of Theatre Goers, a local organisation run, coincidentally, by an old friend's sister-in-law. She organised theatre trips to plays and shows and other excursions, such as a backstage tour of the National Theatre on the South Bank. One memorable trip was to the O2 on a boat built in 1912.

What background music did they play as we embarked? The theme from the film, *Titanic*! Was this a sign of things to come? The guided cruise down river from Tower Bridge was very interesting and, thankfully, uneventful. Of course, Lyn wanted to replicate the scene in which Kate Winslet and Leonardo DiCaprio stood on the bow with their arms outstretched…

After the girls left home, Lyn and I continued to go to gigs; a classic was a Stones gig at Wembley Arena in 2003, a birthday surprise she had arranged for me. This was before she had a mobile phone; she had been out for some time, visiting a friend, and I was getting a little worried. I went out for a while and, when I came back, there was a telephone message to say she was held up. Something had happened to her car and she would be back soon. It was all rather garbled. I did not hear from her for an hour so I asked the operator to do a trace on the number Lyn had called from, which turned out to be a public phone box at Wembley Stadium box office…

I did not know what to do and then she turned up; she was quite upset and said she'd broken down and someone had helped her. I knew by her face that she was telling porkies; she never could lie or tell a fib, it just showed on her face—not a bad trait. I decided not to push it, nor to let her know what I had found out.

It was only months later that Lyn gave me the tickets for the Stones gig, the day before my birthday, bless her. They were great seats about 5 metres from the run-out stage, where the band went to play part way through the gig. I even caught a guitar pick that Ronnie Wood threw.

When we arrived there was a seat next to me that was empty until about ten minutes before the gig started, when a man turned up and, in a heavy Geordie accent said, 'How do. I'm a bit late but I had to finish a job.'

'Ah, OK, so what did you have to finish?'

'I'm an embalmer,' he said, as he took my hand to shake it. I just hoped he had washed his hands!

The theatre was something else that Lyn enjoyed, particularly musicals. We went to quite a few performances in London over the years, including *Hair, Miss Saigon, Blood Brothers and Les Misérables*, which I saw twice with Lyn, while she saw it four times.

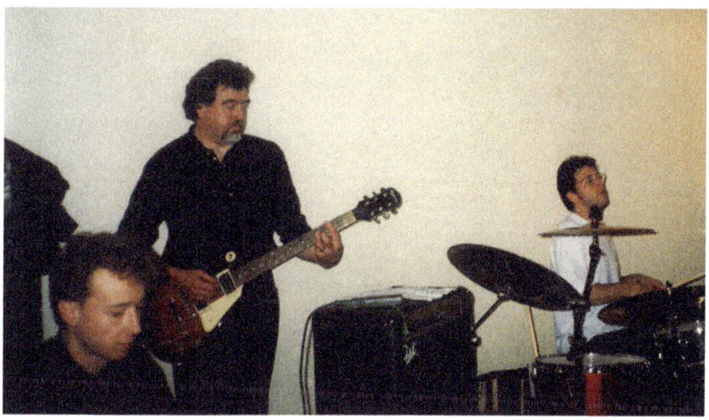

Me (centre) in the band, early days.

12 Our daughters' marriages

Our daughters, Sarah and Kelly, decided to marry in the same year! It was something of a shock, initially, but it made 2006 highly memorable. They had both met their future life partners some years before and been living together for several years. They married their fiancés, Steve and Keith, at All Saints', Harrow Weald, carrying on the tradition for a third generation. Sarah and Steve married in May and Kelly and Keith in September.

Lyn had a few trips, with Sarah and Kelly, looking for wedding dresses, which she loved. The first was a day trip to London to reconnoitre what was available in some of the larger wedding outfitters. She came back exhausted but very happy, having spent the day with her girls. I joined a couple of other trips near where Sarah and Kelly lived; they were equally enjoyable.

Lyn was still using a walking stick at this time, and she was able to fulfil her dream of walking down the aisle at both her daughters' weddings, ably supported by Steve and Keith at each other's weddings, while I walked the girls down the aisle.

We split the costs of both weddings with the girls, their husbands and respective parents, and they managed to stay within the budgets they had set themselves. Both weddings were wonderful and the receptions and evening functions could not have been better, even if you had thrown loads of money at each of them! It is having the family and friends you want with you that makes something memorable, not the amount of money you spend. The services, the receptions and speeches were very special and emotional.

Lyn never stopped smiling, from the morning of the weddings to the time we went to bed; she was where she loved to be most, with her family and friends. I have some great photos of Lyn at the weddings, thoroughly enjoying herself, glass of fizz in hand, and all smiles, just as it should be at your daughters' weddings. There is also a photo of Lyn and her best friend, Chrissie, giggling like two schoolgirls, having had a few glasses of fizz. Both were such special days.

Lyn went on both the girls' hen weekends and thoroughly enjoyed herself, as she had known their friends for several years. I also enjoyed the boys' stag dos.

Sarah and Steve have two children, Matt and Will. Kelly and Keith also have two children, Hayden and Bethany.

There is a saying that your children are a reflection of you; as parents you pass on your own life values to them. I know that Sarah and Kelly and their husbands, Steve and Keith, have passed on those same values to their children. Over the years, I have always felt proud when friends have commented that our children and grandchildren are a credit to us.

Lyn and I had always felt very lucky to have two such caring and loving sons-in- law, who have been such good husbands and fathers, and who I have continued to treat as my own sons.

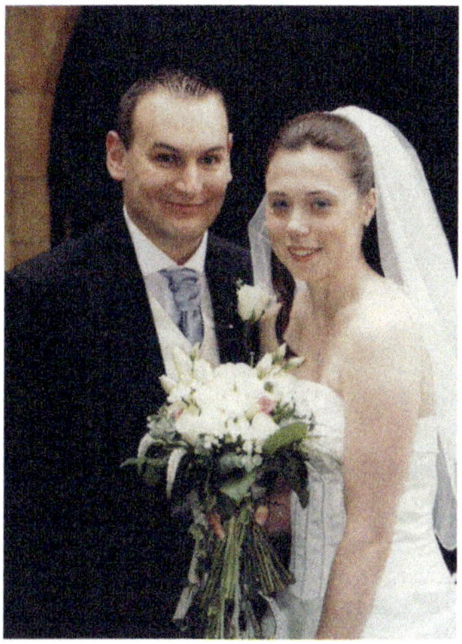

Sarah and Steve,
wedding day.

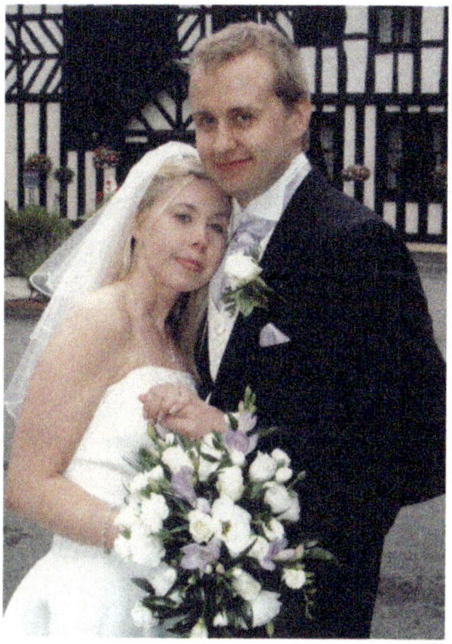

Kelly and Keith,
wedding day.

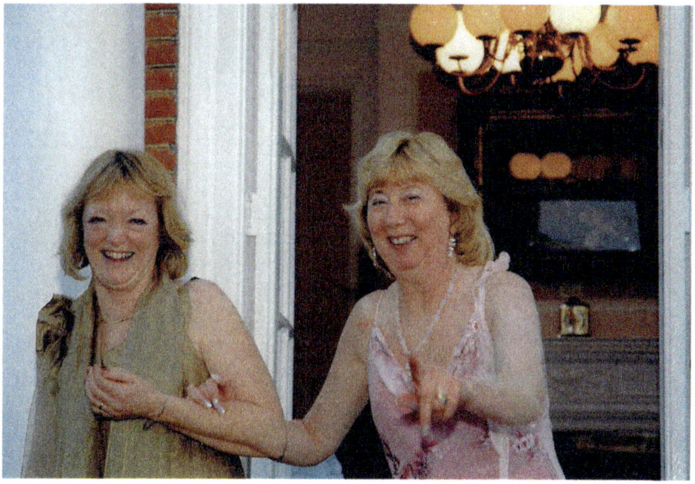

Lyn (right) at wedding reception, with Chrissie.

13 Disability and mobility aids

I cannot remember exactly what year we started looking at aids to help Lyn but it was probably in the mid to late 1990s, while we were in Harrow. First, I fitted some support rails in the shower; at this time Lyn could lift her legs over the bath rim and lower herself into the bath, but she needed a little support from a horizontal rail above the taps to pull herself up. She could also stand and have a shower but needed the support of a vertical rail at the side of the shower valve.

It is difficult enough for anyone, at the best of times, to keep one's balance and operate the shower valve, while standing upright in a shower with water pouring over one's head and into the eyes. For someone with balance issues and feelings of vertigo, it could be disastrous to over-balance and fall. I was always conscious of trying to maintain Lyn's privacy at these times, so I would make sure that she showered and dressed in the mornings before I went to work; I would stay near in case she needed assistance. Maintaining someone's dignity and being ready to help in any situation is a fine line to tread.

In 2000, we built an extension to our house, which gave us some options, with a larger third bedroom upstairs and, downstairs, an additional bedroom/study, a larger kitchen, utility room and a walk-in shower complete with support rails.

There are now so many disability aids on the market and most large towns have a disability centre, where advice is always available on the type of aids a person may need, such as shower grab rails and walk-in baths, for example, or rollators and scooters.

We tried many different mobility aids over the years to help Lyn and make her life easier; simple things like switching to lever taps, as they are easier to use if you have dexterity issues, by simply pushing left or right for hot or cold, and up and down for water pressure, rather than trying to grip a conventional cross-head tap. A fold-down seat in the shower was very useful; when Lyn was feeling tired, even in the mornings, she could sit in relative comfort and wash her hair and shower without worrying about balancing.

It is always best to talk to the staff in these shops, as they deal with all sorts of issues every day and there is probably nothing that they have not come across before. Special aids can be expensive but there are plenty of organisations that can help. It may be that your local MS support branch or even the MS national centre could help with funding via a grant. This is from the MS Society website:

> **MS Society Grants** can be awarded to improve the Health and Wellbeing of those affected by MS and can be used for home adaptations, scooters and equipment. MS Society Grants can also be awarded to unpaid carers for leisure activities/equipment or personal development.
>
> It is also worth getting an assessment from an occupational health therapist through the NHS, they will initially visit you at home to assess what your needs are and they will then arrange that

support for you.

You may be entitled to free home adaptions and equipment provided they cost less than £1000.00 each, for instance:

Handrails for the stairs
Grab rails for the bathroom
An intercom system for answering your front door
Ramps for wheelchair access
A walking frame
Perching stools in your kitchen or shower
Heating system improvements (if it directly affects your medical condition)

The range and design of mobility and disability aids have improved dramatically over the years and there is much more equipment available now to make the lives of people with MS that much easier.

If you need this type of help you should first ask your GP, health professional or MS specialist nurse for an assessment by an occupational therapist, who will come to your home and assess where you live and how you manage your daily life. They may be able to arrange for certain aids to be fitted without the need for any additional funding, so that is the best starting point. If funding is required, I would urge you to contact either your local support group, the MS Society national centre or your local council.

One essential mobility aid that Lyn had from the late 1990s was a car, through the Motability scheme. This enables people with disabilities to lease a car, a wheelchair accessible vehicle, a scooter or a powered wheelchair, according to their individual needs, over a three-year period. To qualify for the Motability scheme, the person with MS must receive one of the following mobility allowances:

Higher rate mobility part of Personal Independence Payment (PIP)
Higher rate mobility part of Disability Living Allowance (DLA)Enhanced rate mobility part of Adult Disability Payment (Scotland)
Higher rate mobility component of Child Disability Payment (Scotland)
War Pensioners'
Mobility Supplement (WPMS)

To qualify you also need to have been in receipt of the benefit before the age of 65, as you cannot claim for Motability after the age of 65.

The dealership or disability shop you choose will have taken an initial deposit down payment, which depends on the vehicle they choose, and make monthly payments for three years using up their DLA. One major advantage of the scheme is that vehicle insurance, annual service costs, tyres and repairs are all covered by the lease agreement; only fuel has to be paid for.

Check the Motability website for details.

You will probably need another important thing—a Blue Badge. This allows you to park in disabled parking bays, which are always located nearer to car park entrances. It can also allow you to park on single yellow lines for up to three hours, provided that there are no loading restrictions.

14 Carers

There is a natural tendency for a family to rally round and care for someone with any kind of disability or impairment; it is human nature. You want to do what you can for your family, your loved ones. If you are new to caring, my best advice is to be wary of taking on too much too soon, especially if you have no experience of being a carer. Your GP or the health professional responsible for the person with MS will be able to point you in the right direction.

Lyn had had to take medical retirement because she was finding it increasingly difficult as her symptoms progressed over the years. I have personal experience only of primary progressive MS—a set of symptoms that can vary, with the individual and become slowly and progressively worse over time. The person with MS and their spouse or life carer may not notice any changes from day to day, as they are often quite subtle, so it is only when you meet someone you have not seen for weeks, months or even years that you might notice a step change.

Lyn was always a positive character; she always wanted to do things that any person without disabilities would do, but she was sometimes confined by her symptoms. Consequently, she relied on me as her personal carer.

There is a saying I heard recently that sums up the bond between the person with MS and their life carer, 'You give each other strength'; that is about right. As the person with MS you gain strength from your life carer; you know they are there to help and support you in whatever way they can, and you gain strength from that. As the life carer, you gain strength from the person with MS, as you know and understand what they dealing with, and you are inspired by their fortitude and inner strength.

There are many people with MS who need care to be provided by care agencies; this is generally where the family either cannot provide the care themselves or because the person with MS needs more intensive or longer periods of care than the family can provide. This can mean full-time, 24/7 care, particularly if the person with MS has secondary progressive MS.

The majority of these agency carers are good, some very good; unfortunately, there are also carers who are unsuited to the role, so they do not do the job properly or with care. They are the people who occasionally end up in the press and tarnish the reputation of all the good carers.

The brother-in-law of a close friend has secondary progressive MS and, recently, their care provider sent a new carer on a shift. He had been in the country for just two days and did not even know what MS is! That was a very serious mistake for the care provider to make; they did not ensure that the carer was experienced and had a knowledge of MS. That mistake could potentially have had some serious consequences, for the person with MS, as well as the care agency.

Whether this is the fault of the council, the agency they employ, or the carers themselves is unclear; reasons seem to vary. One of the main reasons that a care regime fails is a lack of joined-up thinking by the management of some of these organisations. I remember several occasions in Harrow when we had telephone calls from members who had been left in the lurch by their carers. They had either not turned up or were very late, without anyone from the care organisation getting in touch to explain what was happening and why—necessitating many telephone calls by our welfare team to try to sort things out.

There was one occasion when a lovely elderly lady, Olive, who had primary progressive MS and some other conditions and spent most of her day in a wheelchair in her flat, was let down badly by her carers. They would normally start in the morning, get her out of bed, washed, dressed and ready for the day; they helped her into her wheelchair so she could have her breakfast and then get around her flat. She would stay in her wheelchair until they came back to help with her lunch, then help her back to bed for a rest. They would return a couple of hours later and help her into the wheelchair for the remainder of the afternoon, and, finally, pay an early evening visit to help her with her dinner, then get her ready for bed. It all sounds somewhat regimented and she did end up in bed at about 7.00pm, but it was a familiar routine that worked for her and she was comfortable with it. Until one Christmas...

On Boxing Day morning, we had a call from one of our volunteers who had just visited Olive; no carers had turned up at all on Christmas Day and she had not been contacted. She had been left on her own all day and night but did not want to bother us as it was Christmas and she knew we would be with our families. She kept thinking the carers would turn up; they did not and, eventually, Olive went back to sleep until the morning. A very sad, upsetting and horrific incident that should never have happened.

Suffice to say, our welfare team's telephone call to the care company was pretty much one way, direct, forthright and with no punches pulled. The carers were there within an hour. They were very apologetic and promised it would not happen again, but it should not have happened in the first place.

I would like to think that things have changed over the years, but apparently not. I recently learned that one lady with primary progressive MS and other serious conditions had her daily care regime completely upset by her new carers not turning up on time, as the previous ones had always done. The new carers were being sent from one address to another on the opposite side of town, when another team was going in the opposite direction and crossing over. As a result, they turned up at any time of the day. It was a management issue: not having the right people, in the right place, at the right time.

Lyn and I were very lucky to have each other and I was always willing to help with whatever she needed. I will not pretend that it was all sweetness and light; it was not. Sometimes it can be quite difficult, as the person you are caring for can become very frustrated by the whole situation and say hurtful things, but you know they do not mean it.

It was not the same for everyone; there were, sadly, instances when the spouse of someone with MS was unwilling to help them, for whatever reason. As a local branch, it sometimes fell to us to pick up the pieces and arrange for equipment or even carers to come in and deal with things. It was not easy seeing someone with MS suffering without any love and care, and sometimes feeling that your hands were tied.

Below are some extracts from the MS Society's excellent website regarding carers. The website has a comprehensive guide to care services and payments, which will lead you through the steps you need to take to get the best care for you or the person you care for.

> What are Social Care services?
> Social care services come from your local council. They cover all the things you need to stay independent when you have a disability or long term condition like MS. You get these services at home, in the community or in a residential care home. This practical support includes: Information
> Special equipment
> Changes to your home to make life easier
> Someone to help with everyday tasks like getting dressed or washed
> Support for your family carers
> A place in a residential care home if you can no longer live in your own home
> If you are in Northern Ireland social care doesn't come from your council but from Your local Health and Social Care Trust instead. So in our social care information you'll see that we talk about 'your council or Trust'.
> To get social care services, you first have an assessment by your local council or Trust to see what you need. You might have to pay towards the costs of these services. How much depends on your financial situation, and which of the four UK

nations you live in.
On these pages we'll explain how social care could help you.

Why social care is important
What can social care services help with? They help you to stay as active and independent as you can. Social care keeps you part of the community. It can help you hold on to your dignity and quality of life as you face the challenges of MS. Social care can also support the people close to you who look after you. It might be hard to get sometimes. But don't let that put you off asking for it. Social care can make a big difference to people's lives.

The way that the benefits system now works means that anyone requiring a carer can obtain that care in different ways:

The council pays an amount of money direct into your bank account for you to pay for the carer; they will obviously require receipts.
The council arranges your care and pays the provider directly.
A service organisation you choose manages your care budget for you.

So, it may seem that if you pay for your carer directly, you have more control over the service you receive. However, if you do pay a carer directly, you have to assume the responsibilities of an employer, National Insurance,

Income Tax, National Minimum Wage, sickness and holiday pay, pension payments and liability insurance. If you use a care service organisation, it is their responsibility to pay for and maintain the care regime.

There is much to consider so you need to get the best advice possible to suit your individual circumstances. I was talking with a carer recently and she said that the company she works for has a system whereby the carer checks in with a QR code when they arrive to see their client. Before they leave, they have to list on their mobile what they have done that day for the company, so things do seem to be improving in some places.

It would be best to check the MS Society website, or with Citizens Advice, a local Disability Advice Service or other reputable organisation, to help guide you through what can initially be a very daunting and confusing benefits and care system. The bottom line is to discuss your individual requirements with your health professional, or any of the above organisations, to establish what care and help you need before you commit to anything.

Even though MS can take time to develop, depending on the type, as a carer you will find that, over time, you are taking on more and more, not just physical care but also providing support to someone who may also have developed certain anxiety issues. This can increase over time and you are, effectively, like a sponge; you absorb a great deal and, sometimes, you may need support too. Be wary of taking on too much without support from other people with whom you can talk to and share your feelings. You can only take so much without being affected.

Never feel that you are a burden to your family; they

are there to care for you, if they are able to, but sometimes they may also need a little help to help you.

The MS Society offers support and advice to carers, so do not feel that you are alone. The society can also offer help with organising respite care for a person with advanced MS—short-term, complete care designed to give both carers and people with advanced MS a break from the usual routine of caring and being cared for. This allows the carer to have some time to themselves, in the form of additional help at home or a break away. If this is something you could benefit from, as a person with MS or as a carer, it would be worthwhile discussing this with the MS Society.

15 Funding for the MS specialist nurse in Harrow

The MS specialist nurse is an incredibly valuable asset for any community that includes people with MS. It is a role filled by a senior registered nurse who, during their career, has developed an interest in and then specialist knowledge of MS, with many years' experience. They are the link between the person with MS and their consultant; over time they learn as much if not more about the patient as the consultant, but they are able to meet their patients more regularly and, for example, assess individual patients' needs, any changes to their symptoms, any concerns about treatments, if there need to be any changes to medications.

When we lived in Harrow, there was no MS specialist nurse, but there was a clear need for one. Lyn had spent much time with the local MS Society branch in different roles, one of which, as previously mentioned, was welfare. This often involved telephone calls, sometimes late in the evening, from members with MS or their husbands, wives or partners, about different aspects of MS—which a specialist nurse could have dealt with. It became obvious to us that the need for a specialist nurse was going to increase rather than decrease, as there were newly diagnosed members joining the branch quite regularly.

We had got to know the fundraising team at the MS Society national centre over the years, and they were very supportive; they too could see that there was a clear need for that kind of support not only in Harrow but elsewhere in the country. Lyn spent at least a year collating background information, telephoning, emailing and writing to anyone who she thought might help. Lyn and Anne, another branch committee member, had meetings with our GP, the local hospital, local council and the local MP, to try to garner support from anyone who would listen. She even went to the Houses of Parliament, with Anne and some members from other branches, to raise awareness about fundraising for MS nurses around the country. When Lyn got back, she wrote an article for the local newspaper about the visit and the nurse funding campaign. The paper ran a follow-up piece in its next edition and named Lyn as 'an MS activist.' Infamy at last!

There were quite a few instances when some of our members were admitted to the local Northwick Park Hospital for various other reasons. Their MS symptoms and needs were not taken into account when they were admitted, which led to misunderstandings and considerable distress. Lyn managed to contact someone at the hospital to discuss these issues and, accompanied by another member, Inger, gave a talk as an expert patient. It went so well that there were staff not only in the room but also in the corridor outside. Not long after that, the hospital set a process in motion whereby anyone who was admitted and had MS was put in touch with a dedicated nurse with a knowledge of MS. While they might not have been a specialist nurse, at least they had an understanding of the possible issues the patient might be facing and of any additional help they might need. It further underlined the point that, if a specialist nurse had been available, the person with MS could have contacted them. The nurse could then have liaised with the hospital.

Lyn continued to do whatever she could to help with fundraising and, eventually, the MS Society said that they had access to a fund that could provide matched funding—if the NHS would could cover the rest.

Shortly after, Lyn was reading the local paper and spotted an article by Northwick Park Hospital, Harrow about its newly appointed CEO, in which he said, 'Anything is possible' and that he would do what he could to help people locally. Next morning, the first thing that Lyn did was to write to the new CEO to give him a synopsis of the background information as to why a specialist nurse was needed in Harrow. A few days later, she received a telephone call from the CEO's secretary, who said that the CEO wanted to arrange a meeting. As Lyn had collated so much material, she invited him to our house rather than taking everything to the hospital. He duly came to see us; Lyn had all the material piled up on the dining room table and we talked for a good hour about the need for a specialist nurse and how much of a benefit it would be to the local MS community. The CEO agreed that there was a clear need but said that times were difficult and that funding anything was a challenge…

I will never forget the look on his face when Lyn said, 'We have a promise of £60,000 in matched funding on the table from the MS Society for a specialist nurse now, if you can provide the same.' He was understandably taken aback but he agreed to do what he could and promised to get back to her.

A few days later, he was as good as his word and called to say that the funding would be matched. There were quite a few tears of joy and relief that her hard work had paid off after all; her call to the MS Society was predictably well received and the society set about helping to write the brief for the NHS to enable them to start the recruitment process.

So, Harrow now had three years' initial funding for a specialist nurse, which would continue to be reviewed. What did Lyn do next? With help from Anne, she started putting paperwork together to justify the need for another specialist nurse, as one would not be able to cope with the workload in the future! That was my girl.

16 Hot or cold

People with MS have varied experiences of feeling hot or cold. Lyn would always need to keep warm, otherwise she could not function; all her muscles seemed to tighten up, making it difficult to move. In the summer or abroad in warmer weather, she was fine; in late spring and early autumn, she was not too bad, although she would always have to wear or take layers of clothing for any possible eventuality. Late autumn and winter were always the worst for Lyn; when she was outside, she would have to wrap up—again layers were always best.

A few years ago, I bought Lyn a padded pink coat for Christmas, so that was always a staple for her to wear when it was cold; she called it her going out duvet, not a bad description. Even indoors she had to feel warm… We have an oil-fired boiler as we are off the grid for mains gas and we also have an open fire, so we used to have a regular delivery of logs. Between the two heating systems, I was able to keep her warm indoors.

There are excellent gel warming pads that increase your hand temperature, thermal gloves, and even rechargeable heated gloves. Take a look online, you might be surprised but be wary about whom you buy from online; make sure that it is a reputable supplier as, sadly, there are many fake electrical goods, which could be potentially dangerous.

Not everyone was like Lyn; there was one young man—a member of the Harrow MS Society branch—who felt the heat very badly, even when it was cold, to the extent that

I remember visiting him at home in winter and he was dressed only in a pair of boxer shorts!

Everyone with MS is different.

17 Exercise

Exercise for anyone in good health, or any state of health for that matter, is generally a good thing, as long as you do not overdo it but, with MS, it is always worth talking to your doctor or health professional first, if you are unsure, before you do anything.

Any exercise, such as walking, running, jogging, or working out in a gym is good but, with any type of MS, you are limited physically.

Anyone with MS already knows that there are limitations as to what they can do physically; sometimes just moving around the house from day to day. Depending on your level of disability, from waking up in the morning onwards, you are aware of what you can and cannot do. If you were already doing regular exercise and have mild symptoms, you may be perfectly happy to get up and do that or go to a gym to start your day, as so many other people do. It may be that your symptoms have developed and you want to keep exercising but you now feel you can only do it at home. Maybe you are not the sort of person who ever wanted to pound the pavements jogging or go the gym to exercise.

It does not matter what your own personal level of exercise or body movement is, as long as you feel you can get some benefit without overdoing it and making you feel worse, then you are trying to maintain a body fitness level that works for you.

Morning TV programmes and YouTube have classes

that focus on different types of exercise that you can also do from a sitting position in your favourite chair, or even in a wheelchair if that's good for you. Any kind of physical exercise that you can manage without any adverse effects not only makes you feel good physically, it also makes you feel good mentally, which is equally important

Lyn was never a great runner but she ran occasionally for fun and sometimes in a 100 metres competition; I have the photos to prove it. When she could still use a walking stick, Lyn enjoyed walking and so we walked as much as possible within her limitations. In Harrow Weald, there was a large common and woodland open space called Bentley Priory, which formed part of Harrow Weald Common and Stanmore Common. It was near to where we used to live and also had a deer park, an added incentive as Lyn always loved wild animals. We used to go there as often as we could, but sometimes we would just walk around the block at various times of the day, if that was all that Lyn felt like doing. The problem with walking anywhere, particularly with MS, is that you have to keep remembering that, however far you go, you have to return the same distance. Do not overdo it.

There was an amazing facility in Stanmore, not far from where we lived, the Mike Heaffey Centre, now the Aspire Leisure Centre. It was within the grounds and part of the Royal National Orthopaedic Hospital, where it provided rehabilitation facilities for patients, and was also open to the public; you simply joined as a member. There was a fully equipped gym, with many types of equipment; when you joined, the staff would give you a thorough familiarisation session and help you choose the right equipment for your level of disability and they were always on hand to provide help or advice. Lyn was unable to use much of the equipment, but she did use some of the arm-exercising machines and the treadmill set slowly, which meant that she could walk at a comfortable pace, support herself on the frame in front, and stop when she wanted, without having to walk all the way back to the start.

They had one other piece of equipment that was very useful for anyone who could not use all their muscles in the normal way. The Power Plate is a vibrating plate; when you put any part of your body against the plate, it oscillates at up to fifty times a second. This stimulates the muscles in the same way as if you were exercising normally; the micro vibrations activate the muscles, burn calories, improve circulation, and assist muscle recovery.

There was a TV personality, who was paralysed from the waist down, who used to use this regularly when we were there; he would sit or lay on the plate and move now and then, every few minutes, so all the paralysed parts of his body were treated. It is an amazing piece of equipment for anyone with a severe disability. Maybe not for everybody but it might work for you. There are likely to be several gyms similar to the Mike Heaffey Centre, with facilities to suit disabled people; it would be worth looking online to find one near you.

Lyn's main exercise was walking, when she could, as well as using an exercise bike and swimming exercises; like other people with MS, she was limited but she did what she could. The old adage, 'use it or lose it' is very apt; even minimal exercise, if you can do it, is beneficial. Exercise is also very good for your mental health.

From the NHS website:

> It's a scientific fact that regular physical activity and exercise can make us healthier and happier.
> When we're active, the body releases feel-good hormones that can improve our mood and boost our energy.
> Other benefits of exercise for mental health include:
> Boosting our self-esteem and confidence
> Increasing motivation and focus
> Reducing tension, anxiety, stress and mental fatigue
> Helping to calm the mind, especially when dealing with difficult emotions like anger, frustration and sadness
> Reducing loneliness by offering new ways to get together with family and friends and meet new people

The MS Society has an excellent booklet on exercise, which includes:

> Simple exercises for MS
> Symptoms of multiple sclerosis can make it hard to exercise. So we've worked with personal trainer Dom to create a range of exercises for people with MS. These workouts are designed for different levels of mobility.
>
> Pilates for MS
> Research tells us practicing Pilates can help you to manage your MS. It helps most when you practice

often and over a longer period of time. Even doing little or few exercises regularly can make you feel better.

Exercises for MS symptoms

Research tells us exercise can help you manage common MS symptoms, like fatigue, muscle spasms or balance.

We know staying active can:

Help you manage MS symptoms, including fatigue, and problems with balance and walking.

Improve your mood.

Improve your mood when your MS is mild.

Help you to stay as mobile and active as possible when your MS is more severe

Decrease the risk of heart disease.

18 Swimming

In the early 1990s, Harrow's Kingfishers swimming club was set up specifically for people with disabilities; we found out about it through the local MS Society branch. It was based at the Harrow Leisure Centre in Wealdstone, which had a 33-metre pool and a 12-metre baby and toddler's pool. The club had been set up to provide a safe swimming environment, late on Saturday afternoons, when the pool was little used by the general public; a section was roped off for the purpose.

I had been a Borough of Harrow Swimming Club coach at the same pool when our daughters were growing up so, when we found out about it, I was more than willing to go along and provide support for Lyn and any of the other members who might need assistance. I already knew one of the older coaches, who was there as his wife was also disabled. We had access to the floats and other swimming aids, which made helping people with disabilities that much easier.

To begin with, Lyn did have a little more confidence and she was able to swim a short distance with and without a float or help; it was great exercise for her and the other members. One was a member of the local branch called Alan, a wonderful unassuming man, who had been a structural engineer before his MS had developed to the point were he could no longer work. He had a lovely wife, Inger, and a son, Paul. He had cycled to work in London from Harrow and had been a runner—he had even completed the London Marathon in 1985—an inspirational man, if ever there was one.

When I first met Alan, he was in a wheelchair but was still able to get around, I found out that he had never really learned to swim, so I made it my mission to try to help him. Over the space of a few months, we worked together and he started to gain confidence and swim a little with me helping him. This was magical for me as I could see he was enjoying it. Shortly after, Alan became less mobile and began to develop secondary progressive MS, with all that meant in terms of extra care and, for example, more equipment to cope with daily life. But Inger was still very much a driving force in their lives and carried on helping him for several years. Sadly, Alan passed away in 2010.

Another good thing about Kingfishers was that the children of parents with MS or other disabilities could also come along and enjoy simply being together and playing; I know our two girls enjoyed it.

Kingfishers went on for quite a long time but, like many self-help groups it eventually folded through lack of support and funding.

In the early 2000s, Lyn and I used to go to the swimming pool at the Mike Heaffey Centre. It was disability friendly and fully accessible; the changing rooms were either individual cubicles or larger types that were wheelchair accessible, so could accommodate either a family or a person who needed assistance in getting changed. There was a ramped access from the shower area, near the changing rooms, into the pool, and there were handrails all the way down, so anyone who was ambulant disabled could walk easily into the water. The pool also had special wheelchairs that could be used in the water, so transfer into the water for a wheelchair user was easy as well.

Lyn and I went there generally once a week; she was never a great swimmer—like many people of a similar age, her parents had never encouraged her to swim as a child as neither of them could. I was lucky as my dad had taught my brother, Keith, and I to swim and enrolled us at the Harrow swimming club at an early age.

After a while, Lyn had lost some confidence and her MS had started to affect her muscles so we were trying to keep her muscle tone as good as possible. Sometimes, she would use a float to support her arms or upper body and use her legs to move through the water, depending on how she felt. She generally preferred us to hold each other's elbows; I could then walk backwards while she kicked her legs in breast stroke or crawl mode, or she would float on her back, with me at one side supporting her neck and upper body. She never felt out of place as there were so many others with all sorts of disabilities using the pool.

I had also joined an aquaerobics class at the Mike Heaffey Centre; it was a great form of exercise, as it involved exercises like star shapes and moving the knees up and down. We also used polystyrene dumbbells and other shapes using underwater resistance to create the same kind of muscle movements others used with normal dumbbells in the gym. The class consisted of forty ladies of varying ages and me, all supposed to be watching the instructor on the side and following her instructions. There were two ladies in front of me and each week they would chat throughout the entire session, occasionally looking at the instructor and doing a few token exercises. Each time the class ended, one would say to the other, 'Let's go and have a coffee and a chat.'

Lyn did join me once, as she was keen to try it but, even using a swim noodle for support, all the arm and leg movements of forty people in the water made her unbalanced and she felt as if she were drowning. Lesson learned; she never joined a group again, but she was fine doing the exercises if it were just the two of us. For anyone with a disability who can still stand up in water, aquaerobics is a great way to exercise and maintain muscle tone.

Swimming is an excellent form of exercise, as you are using all your body's muscle groups, whatever stroke you use, gentle breaststroke, a more physical front crawl, or even backstroke. Research has shown that thirty minutes of swimming at a steady pace is equivalent to forty-five minutes or more of activity on land. Swimming, like any other exercise is so good for your wellbeing and can help you de-stress, which is very important for people with MS. The repetitive nature of swimming means that you can lose yourself in that zone and empty your mind, or you can use it as thinking time without any external pressures.

19 Trips and their potential dangers

The Harrow MS Society branch bus that I drove for some years was a sixteen-seater, with sideways facing seats, which could be lifted up to allow for wheelchairs. It had been given to the Harrow MS Branch some years before I got involved and was not the most comfortable form of transport—you could almost get a full body massage from a trip…

There were at least twelve members who used wheelchairs and could not safely transfer from a wheelchair in a regular bus so they were the ones who had priority use of the bus. As we could fit only four wheelchairs at a time, it meant no seats so we often needed two trips to collect members from their homes, and back again, for meetings or day trips.

Harrow Council ran a community bus service, which was a great help to so many local groups who needed that kind of transport facility. The buses were better and bigger than ours and could fit four wheelchairs, as well as some seats and, as a local group, we were entitled to two trips per month.

Most of the travel was to Saturday afternoon meetings for a talk or some entertainment; sometimes we would go to an event organised by us or another branch. We once arranged a trip to the London Eye, which also included a riverboat trip on the Thames, before or after, depending on the time of the slot on the Eye. Because of the numbers who booked originally, this proved to be something of a logistical nightmare as we also had to book four council buses. It was not helped when several people withdrew for various reasons and we had to cancel some of the buses. It was, however, a very enjoyable for those that did go.

There is an organisation called the Jubilee Sailing Trust, which in the 1990s had two large full-rigged wheelchair accessible sailing ships, the STS Lord Nelson and SV Tenacious.

Sadly, STS Lord Nelson was decommissioned in 2019.

SV Tenacious was specifically designed for full disabled access and use by a mixed ability crew, aided by the regular qualified crew. Wherever you went on board, the handrails always had an arrow pointing towards the bow so you could never become disorientated.

Every disabled person on board, and any volunteers looking after them, had a chance to sail the ship; the main bridge was set up for full audio-visual control so that people who were partially sighted or blind, deaf or physically impaired, would be able to steer the ship—a tremendous experience for anyone. They even had a wheelchair access lift to a platform part way up the main mast, which meant that anyone with any disability could act as a lookout.

When the last sailing ship Tenacious was being built, we organised a trip to Southampton for a guided tour while she was being finally fitted out. One of our members, Joyce, a lady in her late sixties, was an ardent supporter of the Jubilee Sailing Trust and had been on some trips with them. She was a strong-willed woman, to say the least, and if she wanted to do something she would do it; this led to a few problems over the years.

On this occasion, I wanted everyone to stay together for safety reasons because we were in a large working shipyard. Who went missing at a head count during the tour? Joyce. We searched for her for some time and when I looked outside, I found Joyce after a while in her electric wheelchair, heading down a slipway! The tide could have been coming in at a rate of knots; her brakes could have failed; she could have turned round and toppled over…All these things were going through my head.

'Joyce, what are you doing?' I asked. 'You can't go wandering off in a place like this.'

'I just wanted to see the ships in the harbour,' replied Joyce.

I understood that, but had to give her a telling-off for her own good, bless her.

I recently found out that the Jubilee Sailing Trust charity is going into administration and the Charity Commission will decide its future. Hopefully, something positive will come out of this current problem, as it provided some unique opportunities for disabled people.

20 It's good to talk

All too often, we hear that men find it difficult to talk in certain circumstances. While this may be true for some men, I was always able to talk to my mum and dad about most things, albeit with occasional embarrassment on their part, particularly when it came to sex. But that was a generational thing; I grew up in the 1950s to '70s and there have been major changes in attitudes since then. Lyn and I would talk to Sarah and Kelly about anything when they were growing up and I still do now.

Over the years, going to the local MS Society meetings, I met many people who were newly diagnosed. Most, if not all, of the women who were diagnosed had the attitude of, 'Now I know what I've got, let's find out more about it and see what I have to do to deal with it.' By contrast, most of the men's attitude would be, 'I've got this but I'm the breadwinner, the hunter-gatherer, the family provider. I can't do that now; there's nothing I can do, my life is at an end.' A very difficult, negative and all too common attitude among men, which took a good deal of time to try to change by talking with them.

When you have MS or a similar disease, the best way to understand it and work out how to deal with it, is by talking to people who either have the same condition or are very close to someone with it. Once you know what you have and start to find out more about it and, more important, what you can do to improve things for yourself, the negativity gradually slips away.

There is, of course, much anger and that is totally understandable.

'Why have I got this?'

'Why me?'

'I don't want this.'

'What about my relationship? How will that be affected?'

'What about my sex life, does MS affect that?'

'What about my children?'

'What about my work?'

'What am I going to do?'

All perfectly normal questions and emotions.

It is good to talk and the sooner you do it the better; there are several ways to talk. Our welfare roles with the local MS branch, involved us both in this, often visiting a member who needed help with something, practical help, or passing them on to someone who could deal with benefits issues or carers—but sometimes they just needed to talk. There were occasional night telephone calls; you just had to listen and be a sounding board for someone's anger, frustration, fear even. Thankfully, there were not too many very late calls.

I did not particularly like Lyn dealing with that side of things at the branch, as she also had to care for her own health and wellbeing. But being Lyn, she found it difficult to say no, although I did manage to persuade her not to take the calls if I or someone else could do so.

The main thing is being able to talk to someone; members often found it easier to talk to someone who was known to them but not personally involved and therefore a little detached from the problem, as is often the case in other situations. Just talk; whatever it is that is upsetting, worrying or concerning you, do not let it build up inside you. Like a pressure cooker, you need to open the valve now and then to release the pressure and steam. It is mentally unhealthy to bottle things up; everyone needs to talk.

If you find it difficult to talk to those close to you or if, unfortunately, there is no-one close to talk to, the MS Society offers you different ways of talking—a telephone helpline, as well as online forums and blogs. Choose what suits you best.

21 The pressures on individuals and couples

If someone with a long-term illness or disease is fortunate enough to be in a stable relationship with another person, there is a strong possibility that there will be physical, mental and moral support for that person.

However, I was aware from my very early dealings with the local MS branch that there were some people who had never had a loving relationship or who had been in a relationship that could not withstand the additional stress and strain of dealing with something like MS. This applied to men and women; sometimes it was just too much for individuals to deal with. It is very hard to deal with MS in any relationship; it is also very hard to see someone you love suffer with all the symptoms involved. It is difficult to help a spouse with things they cannot physically do, get frustrated with, and who then takes it out on you. They do not mean to but it is a natural reaction to hit out at the ones who love you most.

When it comes to having help with personal care, such as washing, showering, washing and drying hair, and dressing, the person with MS feels that they cannot fully deal with these things at times. All you can do is to offer help and support when it may be needed. There is a fine balancing act between being supportive and over-protective; simply being there, in the background, when help may be needed is better than constantly hovering and asking if they need help. It is like being on a tightrope and going to whichever side needs to be balanced.

In my experience, it was also very important that I treated Lyn as a woman and helped her feel that she was still a woman, not just part of a disease and a job that needed doing. It can be very easy for someone with MS to feel that they are losing their identity, particularly if the person with MS is a woman; this needs to be reaffirmed and can be done quite simply by continuing to pay her compliments and communicating.

Men with MS can also suffer in the same way but may hide things more; they might also suffer a loss of masculinity (sexual identity), so this needs to be understood and dealt with in the same way for both sexes. Never lose your sense of humour; laugh about the things that always made you laugh, and try to lighten the mood when things are not good.

Some couples that we knew in Harrow did split up because of the strain that MS can put on the relationship; sometimes it would be the husband who left, sometimes the wife; there seemed to be neither rhyme nor reason to it. It is obviously an individual and personal decision. Statistics from a Danish study suggest that MS significantly affects the probability of remaining in the same relationship, compared with the background population.

My attitude, from when we married was that I had signed up for the long haul, 'in sickness and in health, till death do us part,' as the marriage service says. I did not stay merely out of a sense of duty; it never crossed my mind that I would not stay with the woman whom I had loved from the time we met, and help her with whatever life threw at her—and she was the same with me. I believe that support for loved ones and carers of people with MS is as important as treating the patient, and should be understood by health professionals to enable any help and support that their relationship needs to be provided.

It is also worth remembering that you cannot fix everything, so do not try. This is, I think, mainly a male trait; sometimes you just need to listen.

22 Dexterity and co-ordination

Anyone who has MS, or has some knowledge of it, knows how frustrating it is to try to deal with everyday things when you do not have strength or dexterity in your hands and fingers. Over the years, I had to help Lyn with many everyday things as she could not manage to do them on her own.

Opening a bottle

A screw cap can be difficult for anyone. After trying different things, we always had a pair of nutcrackers, which have two different size grips and a pair of longish handles for leverage. This works perfectly; it also works for any type of fizz, as you can ease the cork out rather than letting it hit the ceiling—and losing half the bottle in the process.

Tins with ring-pulls

Tins of baked beans are a classic example. Unless you want to break your nails, on which you might have spent time, effort and money, avoid pulling up the ring with your nails. Instead, slide a spoon handle under the ring and push down against the tin's rim for leverage. Remove the spoon handle, reverse it, then push back against the rim and lift; it works every time.

Buttons

I frequently had to help Lyn with buttons as she could not co-ordinate the fingers of both hands to do up or undo buttons. Clothing manufacturers do not make it any easier by having very little tolerance between the size of the button and the buttonhole.

Bra clips and other similar fastenings

For years, Lyn could not reach behind her to do up a bra, which presented co-ordination and dexterity problems. She used to struggle to do it herself by doing up the fastenings in front of her and then twisting it round the back or 'twizzling', as she called it. She had seen a female comedian on TV describing the process and the phrase stuck; it was convoluted but it sometimes worked. The obvious solution would be what I used to call a front loader, a maternity type of bra where the fastenings are at the front.

Front-fastening bras are now much more widely available, not only for pregnant and nursing women but in the form of sports and post-surgery bras too.

Shoelaces

These are far too problematic in terms of dexterity and co-ordination, so avoid them! Opt instead for Velcro, one of the best inventions. There are now plenty of stylish Velcro-fastened shoes, trainers and sandals available.

Zips

Another no-no; it is very difficult to stand up, maintain your balance, reach behind, hold the dress and zip in different hands, pull up the zip so far—and then reposition your hand over your shoulder and pull up the zip to close it. A difficult manoeuvre even without MS.

Trouser zips

These were also very difficult; Lyn started to buy trousers with elasticated waists that simply pulled up. However, not all clothing outlets sell trousers with elasticated waists, so you might have to shop around or buy online.

Bed linen

The majority of duvet manufacturers fasten their duvets with either buttons that are done up in reverse, so that you do not see them, or the better type—pop studs, which are easier for everyone. These are less common and manufacturers' adverts, packaging or labels never indicate what type of fastenings their products have. I once telephoned a company to ask which duvets in their range had pop studs but, even with some searching, they could not tell me. Maybe this has now changed.

Toothpaste and medication tube seals and caps

Why do manufacturers insist on putting those tiny little foil seals over tubes, which you have to remove after you have taken off the outer cap? I use Voltarol, which has a twist device; you remove the outer cap and place it over the tube. This has a corresponding shaped plastic cap that you then twist off. Simple! Why cannot all manufacturers have something similar? The same applies to the inner cap seals of milk and sauce containers.

Plastic bin liners

Whatever type you use, they are all the same; you have to pull the initial packaging open, then struggle to pull one bag away from the roll. Next, you have to find the part of the bag that separates one side from the other to open it.

Incontinence wash gloves

These can sometimes be an essential to people with MS who have incontinence, but opening the sealed hand wash gloves can be difficult, as the top has to be pulled open, then both hands used to pull apart and open the package.

Packaging

Paper, cardboard and plastic packaging has actually got worse over time. Manufacturers should invite people with co-ordination and dexterity issues to test packaging before putting ideas and prototypes into production. It does not matter whether we have MS or not, at some point in our lives we are all going to face dexterity difficulties with packaging, due to old age. Another thing Lyn always had difficulty with was going into a shop, selecting an item and then trying it on in the fitting room. For some time, this was very difficult for her; the fitting room was not a room, it was at best a cubicle about 1 metre square, so there was very little room to take clothes off or put them on. There is no way you could easily get two people in most fitting cubicles—so that one person can help the other. However, this does seem to be improving and some stores do have larger fitting rooms, so it is always worth checking in advance. For many years, Lyn would have to choose an item of clothing, buy it, try it on at home, then either keep it or take it back to exchange or return it. The pandemic made things much easier for her as she could chose an item online, try it on in the comfort of her own home when it arrived, keep it or send it back. Why did we not do this more, previously?

23 Eating and diet

Lyn enjoyed her food but, like many people with MS, she had to be careful. We generally liked the same food so it was not a problem; our diet consisted mainly of chicken, fish, pasta and rice dishes, fruit and vegetables. Lyn liked most chicken or turkey dishes, roasted or grilled, casseroles and mild curries but she was not keen on darker game birds like pheasant or guinea fowl. Offal was another thing she liked, so we would often have liver and bacon or kidneys and, very occasionally in winter, lambs' hearts; we also liked haggis and celebrated Burns Night every year, either on our own or with friends—haggis, tatties and neeps with a whisky sauce is a wonderful dish.

Although Lyn liked most types of fish—grilled, fried or oven baked—and some seafood like prawns, lobster and, occasionally, crab, she was not keen on what she called 'bottom feeders', molluscs like mussels and clams, which I liked.

Lyn's preferred red meat was lamb, which she loved and, sometimes, pork, but she also liked a steak now and then. As she could never eat a whole steak, we would buy a good quality 200 gram one to share.

We both liked pasta dishes such as spaghetti Bolognese, lasagne, fresh stuffed pasta and risottos, and most fruit and vegetables. If we had chilli, it would generally be made with turkey mince and, very occasionally, minced beef.

It was a well-balanced diet, although Lyn preferred to eat chicken or fish dishes as these were easier for her to digest. MS affected her bowels and she did not like the bloated feeling if she ate something like red meat that was difficult to digest.

We always had to be careful of our eating time; we tried to ensure that we ate by 6.00pm at the latest, otherwise Lyn found it very difficult to digest well before going to bed, particularly if we had eaten red meat. There were occasions when this was not possible and we would have to stay up later than normal to make sure she was comfortable before going to bed.

Lyn did like desserts; she would always work through a menu from the desserts backwards and preferred to have a main course and a dessert rather than a starter and main. When we ate out, she would invariably try some of my starter and eat most if not all of the dessert.

Here is what the MS Society booklet on diet and nutrition has to say:

> Eating is more than just something we need to do. It's something to be enjoyed – it can be a fun social activity, a cultural experience and something to make you feel good. Most people know that eating a healthy, balanced diet is good for your general health and wellbeing. Making changes to your diet can also improve your quality of life and wellbeing. There are many claims about how diet can help you manage your MS, and several special diets have been created that claim to have effects on MS. Some people have reported positive effects from these diets, but it can be hard to know what evidence there is to back up the claims around each

diet. In many cases there isn't strong evidence.

The booklet also looks at the existing evidence to help you decide what to eat.

> We'll also look at the kind of healthy diet that most people should be aiming for – and how to get a balance of the different food groups. Symptoms of MS can sometimes affect what you eat and how you prepare meals, so you'll also find some tips on preparing, planning and clearing away meals. We also provide information of some other organisations that can help with issues around food and eating.
>
> Living with MS is different for everyone. Some people say that certain foods help them, and other people don't notice any difference. But many people with MS say that when they eat well, they feel better. For most people with MS, the best diet is a healthy, varied one.
>
> Some people with MS say that following a specific diet has made a difference to how they feel. Perhaps they have less relapses or it improves their overall quality of life. But other people don't feel this way, and there is little evidence that special diets are a good way to manage your MS. We look at some of the more popular diets that are suggested for MS.
>
> Studies show that being very overweight (obese) when you are a young adult plays a role in your risk of developing MS. While other research shows that 24% of people who live in England and 27%

of people who live in Scotland are obese. Both England and Scotland are in the top 10 of countries that participated in an international survey on obesity. You can lose weight by eating and drinking fewer calories and getting more exercise. Your health benefits most from a healthy, balanced diet. See the NHS choices website for information on losing weight.

So, in essence a varied and balanced diet is also a healthy diet and may have benefits for your MS symptoms.

As always if you have any concerns about your diet you should consult your specialist MS nurse or health professional.

24 Collecting and hobbies

Lyn was a great collector of many things over many years and I have done my fair share of collecting. In our early married years, we collected a few things together, such as glasses and pottery from various places we had visited. Lyn probably bought something everywhere we visited—thimbles, pots, plates, ornaments and so on.

As an avid collector, Lyn was predictably loath to discard anything when our parents passed away, so we also inherited their collections, including a considerable amount of Whitefriars glass. My mum had collected this as they lived close to the Whitefriars factory.

Lyn's favourite things to collect were ladies' powder compacts, mostly Stratton but other makes as well. She had started collecting them about twenty-five years ago when she came across a compact that had belonged to her mum. That sparked her interest and, eventually, her collection ran to over three hundred.

We loved going to antique and collectables fairs around the country, which is where she found most of the compacts, or at her favourite venue, the British Compact Collectors Society annual convention, which we attended for twenty years or so. I made Lyn a wooden display box with a glass lid, which she could use to take a small selection of the best compacts for display; the remainder would be laid out on the table. All the members had a table or two to display their collections and would exchange tales of where they had collected certain items. They used the venue as an opportunity to buy and sell or swap with each other; it was also a chance to meet friends with common interests. Initially, she only needed a walking stick to get around the convention, then her rollator and, eventually, her scooter. Lyn was very knowledgeable about her compacts—their type, design and history—she catalogued them all, and gave talks to local groups like U3A and the local branch of the MS Society. It gave her an interest, something to think and talk about, and enjoy—and it helped to take her mind off the MS symptoms. I still have all the things she collected; they were part of her and us.

We both liked and collected Moorcroft pottery, particularly unusual trial pieces or limited-edition pieces; it is something I still do, as well as collecting guitars, which are my passion.

My girls keep saying, 'What are we going to do with all this stuff when anything happens to you?' The answer is that, long before the time comes, I will catalogue all the good stuff and point them in the right direction to sell it; the rest should go to the local hospice charity shop.

Everyone should have a hobby or interest of some sort, particularly so if you have something like MS; it can very easily help to take your mind off things, even for a little while.

25 Moving house...again

In 2007, Lyn and I started thinking seriously about what we wanted to do with the rest of our lives. I was also concerned that, with Lyn's MS progressing, we needed to consider how we were living and if that could be improved over the next few years. We had always had it in mind to move to the West Country; we had spent many holidays and weekend breaks there and knew some areas very well. So we started looking seriously for somewhere that we liked and a property that worked for us.

Initially, we had looked at a huge area, from Lyme Regis in the east, to Okehampton in the west, and about as far north. Our friends, Chris and Andy, lived in Dulverton on the southern edge of Exmoor and we had visited them over the years, from when their children were quite young. We used Town Mills, a local B&B, as a base and, for three years, travelled around on three or four long weekend breaks, looking at properties.

Predictably, many of them were unsuitable, despite what the estate agents' brochures stated. We wanted a bungalow, near enough to a town or village to walk to or to enable Lyn to use a mobility scooter, with shops covering all our basic needs. Dulverton fitted the bill from the word go, as there was a small Co-op, butcher, baker, chemist, a hardware and other independent shops, a petrol station, three tearooms and cafés and three pubs with restaurants. However, suitable properties did not come on the market that often.

We put our house on the market in 2009, to see what it was worth and to gauge interest; it also allowed us to be able to set a budget for our next home. Chris and Andy kept us in the loop if any suitable local properties came on the market. We did find a couple of bungalows in other towns, which would have worked, and even put in offers but, for whatever reason, we did not proceed much further. We were both great believers in fate, so what would be would be.

We found a bungalow in Dulverton that was ideal, but it was over our budget so we put it on the back burner as, by then, the owners had taken it off the market.

After four months of interest but no offers, we had also taken our house off the market. Then, in early 2010, Chris told us that the bungalow we liked was back on the market—at a reduced price. At about the same time, we had put our house back on the market and there was now plenty of interest.

In March 2010, a few people had looked at our house and we had booked a weekend away to look at more properties in and around Dulverton. On the Thursday, our agents called to say they had had an offer; it was £10,000 short of the asking price but we decided to stick to our guns and said that we would only accept the asking price. We were heading down on the Friday and our agents called to say that the buyer had agreed to the asking price, so we could now go to see the properties, knowing that we were cash buyers, a great position to be in. We looked at four properties that weekend and agreed that the Dulverton bungalow was the best bet; we said we were seriously interested, and we would get back to the agents on Monday. We did our sums and made a cheeky offer, which was accepted. The actual buying process went on for some months but, in August 2010, we eventually moved, to start the next phase of our lives.

Before we moved, we decided to clear out the loft completely and go through everything stored there, to avoid taking things that we would have to sort again. A substantial amount went straight to the recycling centre; some items we decided to keep, others belonged our daughters, so we put them together for the girls to go through and decide what they wanted. The remainder were items that we did not want but that were still in reasonable condition; we thought we might be able to sell them at a local car boot sale.

Lyn was insistent that we wash and iron any clothing items beforehand, which we duly did. When we arrived at the car boot sale, we were given our pitch and set up our two tables, with everything neatly laid out and prices on each item.

A man parked his car by the opposite pitch, opened his boot, laid two blankets on the ground, and emptied four or five big black plastic bin bags full of stuff onto the blankets. Then he stood back and admired his work.

Punters started arriving, took a look at our goods and offered silly prices for items they did not buy. Meanwhile they gathered at the pitch opposite like bees around a honey pot. He sold almost everything, while we sold very little. He strolled over we started to pack up.

'This your first time?' he asked.

'Yes.'

'Ah, classic mistake; you've bought grade A crap… I

brought grade C crap and sold it all for pennies, whereas you've made nothing.'

Lesson learnt; we never did another car boot sale and took all that was left to a charity shop. It had been a very strange experience, wandering around and looking at was for sale; the oddest item was a set of three alloy car wheels—fine if, like Del Boy, you had a Reliant Robin.

The bungalow proved to be everything we could have wanted; obviously, having all the rooms on one level made an immediate difference. The rooms were all of a similar size to our previous house, so fitting everything in was not a problem.

Within days, we found out what a great community Dulverton was; everyone we met was friendly and willing to help us become part of that community.

One thing the garden had was an 11 by 5 metre swimming pool. While this had not been on our shopping list when we were looking for a suitable property, it was a definite plus. I have always been a swimmer, preferably long distances, and as I cannot run due to previous foot operations, it is very good exercise for me. Lyn enjoyed the pool too, with me helping her round, with her holding my arms, as she kicked her legs in either breast stroke or freestyle.

She was also able to use a float or swim noodle on her own and use the polystyrene weights to do some aquaerobics exercises. She used to love floating on her back, with me supporting her underneath her neck while I walked around the pool. Lyn would calmly float, kicking her legs, totally relaxed in her own world.

Shortly after moving into our new home, we started to

change things to make it more suitable for us. I made the main bedroom en suite shower more accessible for Lyn, fitting a low level walk-in shower tray and grab rails to give her support when standing up. We removed a wall to create a large kitchen diner next to the living room and installed a new range of kitchen units.

Not long after we moved in and following a referral from Lyn's specialist nurse, we had a visit from an occupational therapist, who did an assessment of the bungalow— to check that we had everything in place to make Lyn's life easier. The occupational therapist arranged for a shower seat to be fitted, like the one we had in Harrow; this meant that Lyn could shower and wash her hair sitting down, infinitely better than standing up. We also bought a bath seat that Lyn could lower into the water; the beauty of it was that she could sit level with the top of the bath, swing her legs round into the bath and then lower the seat. To get out, she just reversed the process. Brilliant!

It would be six years before we were able to take a holiday. For the first couple of years, we were busy arranging the bungalow the way we wanted, nothing major, just getting things right; this obviously had a cost. Also, the country was still in recession and my work dried up for quite a while; my income shrank and we had to rely on our savings. In 2013, the government introduced the PIP (Personal Independence Payments) system. As part of this restructuring, existing claimants were reassessed over the next few years; all Lyn's benefits were stopped and she had to reapply for everything again, even though she had been on the system for fifteen years. With a lifelong disability she should have been exempt from the process.

It took months to complete the forms, reapply, and then go through an appeals process; she ended up having her benefits withdrawn for over a year until it was sorted out. Luckily, her benefits were backdated once it was resolved.

During this period, Lyn was also looking for something to do in town. The Heritage Centre was looking for volunteers, so she started with one half day a week, working in the shop and showing people around the permanent and topical exhibitions. Being a people person, this suited her down to the ground.

It was so good to have the pool when Sarah and Kelly's families came to stay; the grandchildren loved using it. When we were all in the pool, we would set up a floating volleyball net and have some fun; we would help Lyn to play as well, standing behind her for support so that she could join in. It was so good for Lyn to be able to use the pool as it was excellent exercise, even with her very limited mobility.

In March 2021, it became obvious that Lyn was finding it very difficult, almost impossible, to use the steps to climb in and out. This was something I always helped her with, but it was proving to be too difficult to get her in and out of the pool. There was only one choice—we had to find a way of getting her in and out safely. Several companies provide and install hydraulic chair lifts that lower you into the pool; however, having just come out of the pandemic, it was not easy finding a company that had access to one and was able to install it. I found just one. The company was able to obtain a lift in time to fit it in early June; that enabled Lyn to use the pool for the rest of the summer and autumn until we shut it down that October.

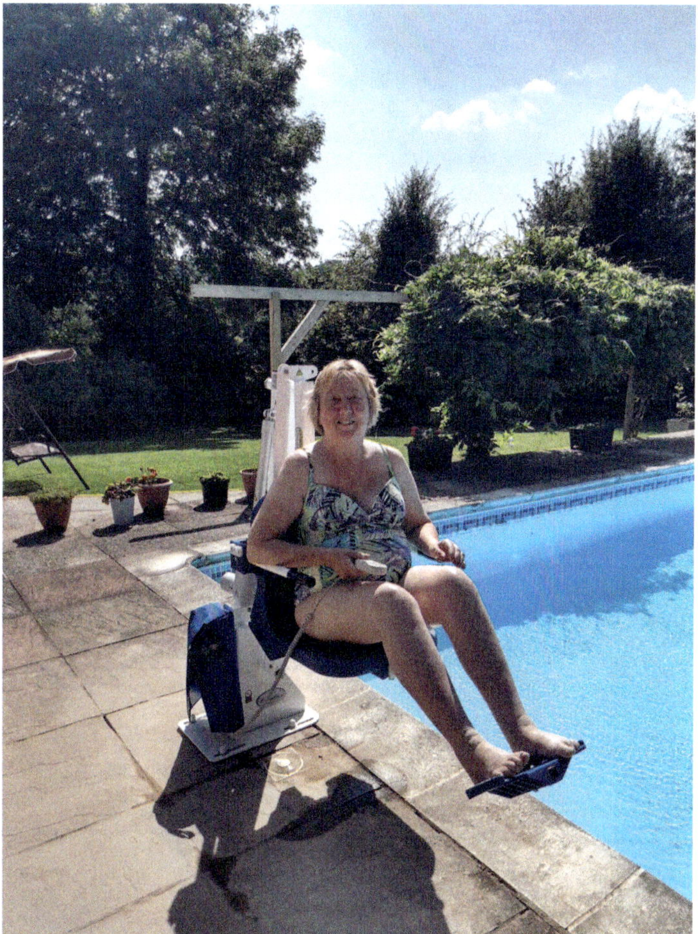

Lyn using the hydraulic pool chair.

26 Holidays

As you would expect with Lyn and her MS, holidays could sometimes be easy to organise, and sometimes difficult or a logistical nightmare, but at least we were fortunate enough to be able to take holidays, which some people could not do.

This chapter includes not only the places we visited but will also, hopefully, give you an idea of what they were like, and where and what is possible, even with a disability.

UK and Europe

When the girls were younger we went either to bed and breakfast for a couple of weeks or to a farm in at Gunwalloe, near Helston in Cornwall, or to stay with our friends, Chrissie and Tim, on their farm in Vimoutiers, Normandy. We also had holidays at other UK destinations and at a couple of Euro-Camps in south-western France, all great fun. The girls loved being on the farms and helping with the animals, as well as playing with other children of a similar age.

When we stayed with Chrissie and Tim, we visited familiar places that we liked or explored new places. Lyn spent many hours catching up with her oldest and best friend, and helping her feed the new calves, while I helped Tim around the farm. He let me drive the tractors and machinery around the farm; for example, picking up feed and taking it from the stores to the cow barn, moving things around the farm, or topping fields.

I once helped Tim with a difficult calving in the early hours of the morning; while he was at the business end, I sat on the straw with the cow's head in my lap, stroking her head and face to try and keep her calm. I will never forget the look of complete trust in her eyes; it was as if she knew I was helping her, an incredible moment I have never forgotten.

Cyprus

In 1994, after Lyn had her hysterectomy, we went on our first holiday to Protaras on Cyprus. As Lyn was recently out of hospital, it was more relaxing than anything else which was just the job.

Italy

In 1995, I booked a long weekend anniversary break in Rome. We visited all the usual sites: the Vatican, Sistine Capel, Colosseum and many more. I had secretly booked a Sunday coach trip to Naples and Sorrento; all I told Lyn was that we were going on a trip and had to be up early. So, we were sitting in reception at 6.45am but by 7.00am no-one had arrived to pick us up; the receptionist, who was in on it, made a phone call, then held up five fingers—five minutes.

Ten minutes later there was a screech of brakes outside and the entrance door flew open.

'Meester 'Ammond, you come quick, we got to go now.'

He ushered us out—to the doorless side of a minibus facing the kerb and walked us to the door opening on the other side. I helped Lyn into the middle seat; the driver had already moved to his seat.

After strapping Lyn in, I strapped myself into the outside seat; the minibus had already started to move, so I reached my hand back to pull the door shut. As I did so, an American voice behind me said, 'It's on the roof; it fell off on the way here…'

'Are we going to Naples in this?' I asked the driver, as we screeched around bends, with me holding on for dear life.

'No, just coach station.'

'Thank God for that,' I thought. We arrived in one piece and had a very enjoyable trip to two of the places Lyn had always wanted to visit.

Cyprus

We returned in 1996 and 1998 and stayed in the same place.

On one of the Cyprus trips, we decided to join a mini two-night cruise to Cairo, as it would be a chance to see the Pyramids, the Sphinx and the Egyptian Museum in Cairo. It was very interesting, but there was no way that Lyn could clamber down into the depths of the Great Pyramid; she was also a little claustrophobic, so only Sarah and I went inside; Kelly stayed at ground level to keep Lyn company. At some point, Lyn decided she wanted to mount a camel and went for a short ride. She was game to try things, so why not? The camel driver asked for money to let her dismount, which I declined, and he headed off to the Egyptian Tourist Police, who were always around…Lyn was screaming to be let down. I knew he would fear being arrested for abduction so, after a few minutes standoff, he let Lyn dismount.

On our last family trip to Cyprus, we had hired a

four-wheel drive Rav 4 to tour the island, particularly the Troodos Mountains, which had spectacular scenery. We once stopped for a picnic at a bay by Aphrodite's Rock, near Paphos. There is a local legend that if you swim three times around the rock you will meet the love of your life and increase your fertility. I was not that bothered by this as I had already met the love of my life and long since had a vasectomy...

It is known that the currents around the rock are quite strong—but I was a strong swimmer. I swam round it once so that Lyn could take a photo of me through the hole at the base of the rock. When I had swum back to shore, Lyn said, 'Could you do it again? I couldn't see you!'

Sarah and Kelly went back on their own in 1999; they had a great time, but there was something of a scare when Kelly became dehydrated and ended up in hospital for a night and day. Fortunately, Sarah was able to pay with a credit card on my account and we contacted some friends, Lynn and Darren, who lived nearby, so the girls had some adult help!

During those 1990s holidays, Lyn's MS had developed but quite slowly; there were times when her balance was an issue, but she was able to walk with my support and with a walking stick as necessary. At about this time we were beginning to accept that the idea of long-haul flights might not be possible at some time in the future. We did not know how long Lyn would be able to cope with them as her MS progressed. In 2000, we made the conscious decision to visit as many countries as we could afford to over the coming years, for as long as possible.

Lyn was a member of the Civil Service Motoring

Association and, even though she had retired, she could still retain her membership. The CSMA produced a monthly travel magazine and always had adverts for different holiday deals; the first offer we responded to was a trip to Borneo.

Borneo 2000

A holiday in Borneo had been a long-held wish for both of us—to experience the country and see the wildlife. Sarah had decided to come with us as she was also keen to see Borneo; Kelly was less interested in visiting the jungle and was quite happy to have the house to herself for a few weeks and spend the time with her boyfriend, Keith.

The outward flight had a stopover in Singapore for a few hours and we stretched our legs. In Borneo, we stayed at Kota Kinabalu on the north west coast, a delightful place; the resort was welcoming and the local people were too. We were on a fifteen-day holiday and stayed at the resort for five days, chilling out on the beach and around the pool. Next was a trip to the other side of the island which involved two internal flights, multiple minibus rides, a two-night stay at a river lodge, river cruises, more minibus rides and a boat trip. With so many things involved, it could all have gone horribly wrong at any point, but it did not.

Mercury, the holiday company, organised the trip and minibus journeys and Malaysia Airlines the flights. If they said we were leaving at 8.00am, we left at 8.00am; if the boat was due to leave at 10.00am, it left at 10.00am. Disability access help had been organised at every stage of the trips and was there when needed, be it a wheelchair or a lift onto the aeroplane. They were brilliant and nothing was too much trouble; if one thing had not happened on time, it could have ruined the whole trip, but nothing went wrong; it was faultless.

For the rainforest trip, we took an early flight to Sandakan on the north east side of the island. The first stop was at Gomantong, one of the biggest caves in the world, where they still used to collect birds' nests for soup from the roof, about 30 metres above us. Amazing, but the smell of ammonia from centuries of bat droppings on the cave floor was overpowering. There was one quite tense moment when I had to quickly pull Lyn's hand away from a whip scorpion on a support railing; they can give a nasty—but not fatal—nip.

In the afternoon, we visited the orangutan reserve at Sepilok and saw the orangutans in their natural habitat; first, orphaned babies, which were unbelievably cute, then juveniles and adults outside the orphanage area. They kept the orphans for the minimum possible time and gradually released them into the rainforest. They were only fed bananas, to bore them with minimal choice and to encourage them to explore and find more exciting food in the rainforest.

We then had a two-night stay in a river lodge with two daytime trips on traditional riverboats to observe wildlife from the river, rather than trekking through the rainforest, and two days' cruising, taking in the views and taking photos of the abundant wildlife. We met a man travelling solo in a boat, apart from a guide; he was a freelance photographer working for National Geographic, on a three-week assignment taking as many photos as he could.

He told us that National Geographic would probably publish only three or four in the magazine—what a life!

A trip to Turtle Island in the Sulu Sea followed, to see a turtle lay her eggs on the beach at night. We were called in the late evening and watched her lay them, with tears in our eyes; it was one of the most emotional things we had ever witnessed and the trip culminated in releasing newly hatched baby turtles into the surf first thing the next morning. All in all, an amazing experience and one which Lyn and I never forgot.

We returned to the resort for another week of chilling out. Disabled access in the resort was very good; outside was a little hit and miss and many pavements were up and down, so not suitable for a rollator or wheelchair. Lyn's MS was still slowly progressing, but she definitely felt the benefit of the warmth, although she did sometimes feel the effects of the humidity.

After relaxing for a few days, we decided to go parascending over the South China Sea, Lyn was a bit wary at first but once she was on the boat ready to go she loved it.

On the way home we had also booked a two-day stopover in Singapore, where we visited the botanical gardens and took a cable car ride to Sentosa Island. We had afternoon tea at Raffles Hotel, which was quite an experience, and a Singapore sling in a rooftop bar overlooking the city.

USA and Niagara Falls 2001

I had a friend, Robert, who had moved to the USA for work; his company had offered him an eighteen-month contract with his company, setting up a manufacturing plant in Weston, Massachusetts—near Boston—so he and Fiona decided to take the opportunity and move with their family for the experience. They had been there for a while and invited us to stay with them. We booked a fly-drive trip and spent three weeks using their house as a base, while travelling around New England.

We had arrived late in the afternoon and Lyn was feeling rather travel sick. Robert was going to pick up a Chinese takeaway meal and there was a pharmacy next door. While Robert collected our meal, I went to the pharmacy, where a young Chinese American lady was behind the counter; I told her that my wife was feeling a bit sick.

'A bit sick?'

'Yes'

'Sick, is it food?'

'No, she just feels a bit sick after travelling.'

'So not food?'

'No.'

'But what? Why she feel sick?'

'She just feels a bit queasy.'

'She eaten gweasy food?'

'No, no, not greasy food, not food at all, she's just travel sick. Have you got any Milk of Magnesia.'

'Yes.'

'OK, I'll have that, thanks.'

Job done.

When I met Robert in the car, I told him what had happened.

'How the fuck did you expect her to understand "queasy"?'

Fair point.

We visited many places in New England and even went on a whale-watching boat trip from Cape Cod, where we saw some humpback whales. The highlight of our holiday was a three-day trip to Niagara Falls, which I had organised for Lyn's birthday. Part of the experience was a river trip on a boat called Maid of the Mist, which went right up to and under the spray of the falls; there was so much water spraying around that we were all supplied with kagouls. The most memorable thing was looking at Lyn, the water running off her hood, and seeing the tears of sheer joy running down her cheeks at being in that magical place on her birthday—an image I will never forget.

Wherever we went in the USA, we found the food portions for any meal so large. We could not eat that much so we eventually decided to order one meal only and share it. For instance, a surf and turf meal in the UK will be a four to six-ounce steak and a few king prawns; in the USA it would be a twelve-ounce steak and a lobster!

If we had not finished our meal, we were invariably asked if we wanted a take-out box…But when you are travelling what are you going to do with leftovers? We never bothered.

On the Sunday morning we left Niagara, we had a 450-mile drive back to Weston so, after we had finished eating breakfast, we piled up a plate of pastries and croissants and asked the waitress for a takeout box.

'Sorry, we don't do those at the Sunday breakfast buffets.'

The one and only time we needed one!

We explained where we were going.

'Leave it with me,' she said.

A few minutes later, she came back with a large

aluminium foil bag full of the goodies.

'There you go.'

Hospitality at its best.

There were some long drives on that holiday, particularly from Niagara to Weston, up to New Hampshire and Vermont and then to New York for the flight back home; fortunately, there were plenty of toilets along the way. Disabled access across the parts of USA we visited was generally very good.

Egypt 2002

Never happened…

On a Friday, a few days before my fiftieth birthday, Lyn felt very rough. She had not been well the day before; now she was in a lot of pain and needed to see a doctor. We managed to get an appointment. After examining Lyn, the GP said, 'I'm going to call Northwick Park Hospital and book you in; you should go there now.'

'Why?'

'I think you have a serious problem with your gall bladder.'

We got into the car and made our way to the hospital.

'Well,' said Lyn, when we were on our way, 'you were going to be packing the suitcases tomorrow; now you'll have to cancel the trip.'

'What trip?'

'I had booked us on a mini cruise down the Nile to look at ancient Egypt for your birthday; we were to fly out on Monday.'

Lyn was checked in at A&E and hospital staff took her quickly to the X-ray department, before settling her in a bed on a ward. I went to the hospital the next morning, just as the doctor arrived. He said that Lyn's gall bladder looked like Brighton beach; there were so many stones and it was on the point of rupturing. Lyn had her gall bladder removed later that day.

I shudder to think what would have happened if we had been on board on the Nile when that happened. All ended well and we managed to get the money back on the travel insurance.

Barbados 2003

The first time we went to Barbados was, again, through a CSMA magazine deal. Most people assume, quite wrongly, that you have to spend £10,000 to £15,000 a week to go to an all-inclusive, gated resort in Barbados. We stayed for a week at a fantastic little resort, a mile or so inland near Speightstown on the west coast. It consisted of no more than twenty bungalows, dotted around the gardens and a swimming pool; each had a bedroom, shower, a living-dining room, a kitchenette and a patio. We paid £800 for the two of us for bed, breakfast and evening meal and the return flights were £400 each; a very good deal for somewhere like that. They had a regular shuttle bus every hour that would take you either to the town or the beach and then pick you up. What a wonderful place and wonderful people. We met many local people; some have remained friends ever since.

Disabled access in Barbados is good in the main towns and shopping areas, hotels and tourist spots; however it can be a bit hit and miss in the smaller towns, as the pavements are uneven. The same applies to many main roads, so access by wheelchair and rollator can be difficult, if not impossible.

Australia 2004

On our first trip to Australia, we did a three-week, part fly and part coach trip; we stayed at each stop for two days, starting with a two-night stay in Perth, and then flew to Alice Springs in the Red Centre. When we arrived we just had time to check into the hotel before we went by coach to see Uluru (Ayers Rock) at sunset, while having a barbie and a glass of fizz; an amazing sight. It was only slightly topped by going back before dawn the next day to see the spectacular sunrise, but just coffee this time.

While we were in the outback, another highlight was an air balloon ascent at dawn; we arrived in the dark at about 4.00am and spent some time getting the balloon and basket ready, then took off just as the sun was rising. Flying above the birds and seeing the wildlife just starting to move was spectacular. It was slightly difficult to get Lyn up and over the basket sides but we did it, with some help, and it was worth the effort she needed to do that. You just have to try these things; there is always a way.

After we had landed, we went for breakfast but Lyn said she needed to go to the toilet and asked where to go.

'Well, there's a bush over there for the boys and there's a dunny behind the other bush for the ladies,' was the reply.

Lyn went with another lady for company; the dunny was a huge pot with a seat and a proper toilet lid, which Lyn lifted. It was empty except for a lizard at the bottom. Lyn screamed, shut the lid, and they opted for the bush instead.

The breakfast was a barbie; barbecued chicken and sausages at 9.00am was a first. That evening, we went to another barbie by a dried-up riverbed; great food and beers. I innocently asked our host if the river ever flowed in the wet season.

'Yep, it did a few years ago, ruined the annual Alice Springs Yacht Club boat race.'

'What? How?'

'Well, every year all the teams race by running down the dried-up riverbed, with the boats over their heads. They couldn't do it with the river flowing; buggered it up completely.'

I love Aussie humour.

We then travelled to Cairns in Queensland; we were there for three days, so we hired a car to drive around and visit places as the mood took us. We went to a working crocodile farm, where we had a close-up view of the crocs—from a boat on the lagoon—at feeding demonstrations. The crocs leapt up, almost their entire length out of the water, to snap at food.

One day, we visited the Great Barrier Reef; the boat took us to a pontoon and from there you could go underwater in a submersible, which Lyn did and loved, as she was not a great swimmer. I took the opportunity to go snorkelling. There was an amazing number of fish and the reef was spectacular to swim over.

We then flew down to Canberra, Australia's capital and political centre, but only passing through for one day. That was, frankly, more than long enough as it is probably the most boring place in Australia.

Sydney was the next stop on the coach drive; we went on the obligatory harbour cruise, which was excellent as it took us all round the bay, which was spectacular. We also visited other sites around Sydney.

Our next stop was Melbourne, where I had some friends, Tim and Pat. I first met Tim at secondary school and we had stayed in touch on and off over the years, although more so since the early 2000s, via email. After our two-day Melbourne tour, we stayed with Tim and Pat for a week and they showed us more of Melbourne's surrounding areas.

Disabled access: pretty much everywhere in Australia is disabled friendly and accessible; the only exceptions would be in very small locations in the outback.

Bangkok

On the way home from Australia, we had a three-night stopover in Bangkok, Thailand, and had hired a minibus for two days' sightseeing, with a driver and guide. On day one, we drove around the city looking at many temples, palaces and statues of the Buddha; there are so many that we would never have seen them all.

On day two, we drove out to the jungle to Kanchanburi and visited a museum devoted to World War II and the Japanese occupation. We managed to get Lyn into a traditional river longboat—James Bond style with a car engine on the back and a long prop shaft—and sailed up the River Kwai to the famous bridge. Hair-raising to say the least, but we made it in one piece. I was sitting at the front and, when I turned round, Lyn's face was a picture: trepidation, fear and exhilaration all at once, but she loved it. Because of its history, seeing the bridge at Kwai is quite emotional; there is a museum, which tells the story of the death railway. The current bridge is not the original timber version built by prisoners of war (and which was shown being blown up in the film); that was destroyed by allied bombing; it is a concrete and steel bridge built by Japanese engineers and Allied prisoners. It was repaired after the bombing and its still in use today.

That two-day minibus hire, with a driver and guide, was about £100 for the two of us; at the time, you could have spent more than that going round London in a black cab for less than a day.

Disabled access around Bangkok was inconsistent; the hotels, large buildings and shopping centres were better, but most pavements, even on main roads, were not good. We had to walk in the roads, which was very tricky, so we did little walking.

Morocco 2005

A pleasant two-week holiday in Agadir, relaxing and chilling by the pool, was just what we needed at the time; the resort and surrounding areas were very accessible for anyone with a walking disability. We occasionally took a cab into the city and visited Marrakesh, which was amazing, also Essaouira .

Barbados 2006

We went room-only this time, as we had found out on our first trip that you could buy good food at the local supermarket and fresh fish markets, at reasonable prices. This was great as you could simply cook what you wanted, when you wanted and, if you fancied a meal out, there were plenty of restaurants to cater for every budget.

One day we went on a catamaran cruise; we were

cruising for about half a day, looking at the ocean and land views; there was an opportunity to go snorkelling, which I could not resist. Captain Ahab—yes, that was his real name—said that Lyn could stay with him on a deck that was lowered to just above water level. She had as much fun doing that above water as I had under water; she even had a turtle feed out of her hand.

Minorca 2006

Another chilling holiday for a week, to get some warmth in Lyn's bones; the island was delightful and was generally accessible. We generally stayed in the resort, as we were relaxing; we hired a car one day and managed to drive round the whole island, stopping at a good many places.

Caribbean Cruise 2007

On our previous Barbados holiday, we thought about visiting one of the other islands but it was not possible. The islands collaborate to make their tourism industry work so, if you wanted to fly to another island, the regular flight was at 4.00pm. To make sense of the trip, you had to stay overnight, so that you could spend most of the following day there. We could have hired a private charter plane or boat but that would have been prohibitively expensive. The compromise was a cruise; neither of us particularly liked crowds of people around us but we managed to find a 'cruise for people that don't like cruising.'

The cruise lasted two weeks, starting in Barbados and visiting St Lucia, Dominica, St Kitts and Nevis, St Martin, Antigua, Martinique, St Vincent, Grenada, Tobago and Isla Margarita, off the coast of Venezuela. We visited each island on some sort of trip by coach, taxi or railway, for example, even walking at times, and they were all highly enjoyable. The people we met were delightful and the trips definitely gave us a flavour of the other islands. The oddest thing we saw was on St Martin, where the planes flew in to land only a hundred or so feet above the beach at the end of the runway. Absolutely bonkers!

Even though there were only fifteen hundred people on board the cruise ship—small compared with what was then the average, two to four thousand people—it was still too crowded for us. Some of today's cruise ships are larger.

In terms of disabled access, all the Caribbean islands we saw were the same. Around the streets in the main towns it was fine, but pavements could be challenging

Sri Lanka and the Maldives 2008

Sri Lanka

In 2008, we went to Sri Lanka for two weeks and stayed in Kalutara, about half way down the west coast. Another wonderful place but our first visit involved a six-hour drive from the airport in Colombo along the coast road. The first thing you notice on a coach drive is that there are rules, but only the local drivers seem to know them. I thought that navigating London's Marble Arch and Hyde Park Corner roundabouts was intense; you had to know exactly where you were going and had to get in the right lane at the right time for your exit. Anyone not knowing what they were doing could end up going round in circles for some time. But the main roundabout in Columbo was something else entirely; the drivers just drove straight out, no signals, lots of horns blaring, headed to where they were going. We experienced that roundabout and others fairly often on various visits; the first time you just shut your eyes and hoped the coach reached the other side; once you were used to it, you simply accepted the status quo and trusted that you would, somehow, get to the other side.

The main road to Kalutara was also something of an adventure; there were two lanes that drivers managed to turn into five, normal traffic, such as cars left and right going in opposite directions, beyond them—between the road and what passed for a pavement—were the tuk-tuks, while, in the middle, was a self-imposed lane used by buses, coaches and lorries, which moved along at a rate of knots. When something came the other way, they just eased into the normal lane; the other drivers moved over a little and, when they had passed, they went back to their normal positions. An eye-closing moment to start with but, eventually, you learned to accept that you would reach your destination.

The hotel was called Tangerine Dreams; it was slightly run down but it was clean and tidy, set in its own grounds by the beach, with a pleasant pool. The staff were very attentive and the grounds were spacious, with plenty of trees and plants. It also had the advantage of a having a health and wellbeing spa, which was what first attracted Lyn to the hotel, as she loved having different massages and reflexology. I like a good massage too, so we spent a good deal of time using the hot tub and having massages.

One memorable day, there was a wedding at the adjoining hotel; the exquisitely dressed bride and groom arrived on equally elegantly decorated elephants. Not the sort of thing you see every day.

The hotel, like most others, had lifts to all floors and the paths and grassed areas in the gardens were all accessible. Outside the hotel, there were no pavements as such, so using a rollator or wheelchair could be a bit hit and miss.

The Maldives

On the way back from Sri Lanka we had a four-night stopover on an island called Meedhupparu, in the Maldives. The only way to get there was by speedboat or seaplane from the main island of Mal; we opted for the seaplane—what an experience that was.

For many people, the Maldives are the dream holiday islands: sun, white sand beaches and clear blue water. Lyn enjoyed the warmth, although we were often in the shade as the sun was just too intense for comfort. I did plenty of snorkelling over the reef, where there were so many different fish to see. As the water between the beach and the reef was so flat and calm and the seabed was shallow sloping, Lyn often joined me in the sea and even tried snorkelling. On one occasion, we had some manta rays swimming around us; they were so slow and gentle that Lyn was just happy to let it happen—magical.

Sri Lanka 2009

We returned and had the same enjoyable holiday at the same hotel—but with more massages.

Barbados 2010

Another two-week holiday for a warm break from the cold UK; just the job.

France 2016

We stayed with our friends Chrissie and Tim in Vimoutiers again; a lovely break and a chance to catch up after a long time.

Kerala 2017

For the first four days, we were on an organised tour, spending the first day and night aboard a converted rice barge on the rivers and canals that were once used for transporting rice. The second day was a wildlife reserve safari, where we stayed overnight. As with most safaris, you never seem to see the big cats, but it was still enjoyable as we did see other animals. The next day we went on a dawn boat trip around the lake to watch all the animals, elephants, different kinds of deer and others come down for their morning drink and to swim. With the mist still clearing as the dawn light changed, it was a magical sight.

The rest of the holiday was spent at a hotel in its own grounds, with a pool by the beach and a spa for more massages, although we did take a tuk-tuk to some local beaches. A wonderful place with wonderful people. The entire hotel grounds of the hotel were accessible, including level paths and a lift. Immediately outside the hotel there were some level pavements and pathways, which Lyn managed to get round using her rollator. But it was a different matter a short distance away; most of the roads did not have any pavements, so disabled access was not really possible.

Koh Samui, Thailand 2018

A wonderful island; we stayed at a beach resort with a

series of single storey cottages that had a bedroom-living room, a bathroom and a shower open to the sky, which was amazing in daylight and under the stars. There was a restaurant and bar on the beach. It was delightful, with a pool by the beach, and I even managed to get Lyn onto the beach and into the sea. This was not always easy, depending on whether the beach was level or if there was a shelf below the waterline, and what the water movement was like.

The best thing for Lyn was the massage spa which she took full advantage of; she loved a relaxing massage—reflexology, a back and neck massage, or a more intensive Thai massage. I would go snorkelling while she relaxed in the spa.

We always seem to meet different people on holidays; some you connect with and you stay in touch. These included some new Aussie friends in Koh Samui: Kim and Trevor from Adelaide, with whom we spent a good deal of time.

The entire resort was on a slope, with paths running everywhere, so it was fine for able-bodied and ambulant disabled people but, even though Lyn took her rollator, it was not particularly easy. However, they had quite a few golf buggies, so you could just call reception, ask for a lift, and they would take you wherever you wanted to go in the resort. So, access across the resort was not an issue.

Majorca 2018

We went on a one-week holiday to a resort called Puerto Pollensa in north east Majorca, a delightful place, with an excellent hotel right by the sea. We had found out about the resort from our daughter Sarah, as she had been to the area several times. Everywhere was flat, particularly the pedestrian area next to the beach, which led to the town and was totally accessible. I managed to hire a scooter locally, in advance, for Lyn, which was kept in the hotel luggage room; this meant that we could easily explore the resort and town.

Australia 2019

We decided to stay for a while with our Adelaide friends, Kim and Trevor, and then go on to Melbourne to stay with Pat and Tim—before flying up to Brisbane and embarking on a 2000 kilometre drive all the way up the east coast, stopping at pre- booked hotels in towns. Predictably, Lyn was concerned about the location and number of toilets on our route. However, I discovered online that someone had kindly produced the National Toilet Map of Australia; there were more than enough and many also had showers. The trip lasted two weeks and we stopped in some amazing places.

At one stop, we took a boat trip to Fraser Island, which, at 120 kilometres long is the world's largest naturally formed sand island. We took an island tour in an air-conditioned, four-wheel drive bus, visiting the rainforest, a crystal clear inland lake, and the wreck of a ship called the Maheno, which was beached in 1935. Part way through the trip, we were offered the chance to take off from the beach in a six-seat plane and fly over the island back to the start point, rather than going back on the bus. We had to say, 'Yes!' With some help from the pilot, we managed to lift Lyn into the cabin, next to the pilot, where there was more room, so she had the best views and photos.

Some days later, we took a boat trip to the Whitsunday Islands. The captain told us that they had been raising money for something they had just fitted for disabled passengers to use on the beach. When we arrived at the beach, he asked us to hold back till everyone had disembarked; then he led us onto the lift platform at the stern and helped Lyn into a wheelchair with huge balloon tyres. Brilliant—I could push her anywhere, even on the soft sand. We played in the shallow surf for a while as the wheelchair was so light that it could float, which was fun for Lyn; thankfully, it did not turn into a Del Boy moment, with Lyn drifting off out to sea. The crew took some promotional photos of Lyn in the beach wheelchair, which they planned to post online to show that disabled people can access remote beaches. We spent a good few hours there and had a picnic on the beach. I did some more snorkelling; this time, we all had to wear very thin skinsuits that protected us from jellyfish.

The final stop was Cairns, where we spent three days exploring. We had a great day trip to the Daintree Rainforest, which started with a very interesting visit to a First Nation Aboriginal cultural event. We then went up to the rainforest on a skyrail cableway; the scenery below was stunning and we rode back down on the historic Kuranda Scenic Railway.

Our last full day was spent on the Great Barrier Reef. What an amazing place; we had been there before, but it is always exciting to revisit. When we reached the pontoon over the reef, we decided how to spend our time. I love snorkelling, which Lyn could not do, so she went on a trip in a submersible. I joined a resident marine biologist and a small group of experienced snorkellers over the outer reef, rather than in the roped-off area immediately around the pontoon. The fish and other sea life were stunning. At one point, we swam over a couple of sharks about 10 metres below us; our guide pointed down and gave the OK sign with his thumb and forefinger and carried on over them. I thought that if it was fine with him, why should I be worried? Lyn was equally happy seeing everything from the safety and security of the submersible.

Back on the pontoon, we had a terrific barbie lunch and noticed a small helicopter on a pontoon a little way off; we found out that they were making a trip over the reef...Did we go? Absolutely! With opportunities like that, you are never sure if you will ever visit again, so you have to grasp what is on offer with both hands and go for it. There were six of us on the trip; it was huge fun and we took some great photos.

Barbados 2020

This was our last holiday together; we flew out on 7 February and returned on 21 February. A month later, the UK was in its first full lockdown due to the Covid-19 pandemic. I am so glad that we managed to take that holiday before the pandemic restrictions, and also before Lyn passed away, as there were few opportunities between 2020 and 2022. At least we had that last time together in the sun and warmth, in a place we both loved; we even caught up with friends we had made over the years.

We had booked into a small development of three

apartments around a garden with a pool in the middle. It was so good to see Lyn relaxing in the sun or swimming in the pool with me. She had not been able to go into the sea in Barbados as it was either too rough or the beach shelved down too much.

We did one new trip, on a boat out to sea for a few miles and then down in a submarine; we managed to book the front seats, just behind the pilot. Lyn loved seeing all the different fish, from angelfish to sharks, and other sea creatures in their natural environment.

We visited all the usual haunts that we had been to before: the beaches, the east coast at Bathsheba, the Round House for a never to be missed Sunday lunch buffet, the rum distillery at St Nicholas Abbey, and the shops, beach bars and restaurants around Holetown and Speightstown. In the evenings, we went to the Little Bristol Beach Bar in Speightstown to see some bands play.

I have a special photo of Lyn at the Fisherman's Pub in Speightstown, dancing one lunchtime to some great reggae and soul tunes, lost in her own warm, happy, small place in the sun.

We were very lucky to be able to have these holidays and I do not regret spending the money, as it was what we set out to do—visit as many places as we could, while we could. Lyn enjoyed every minute, which was what it was all about, building memories...On all these travels, Lyn could get around either with a walking stick, her rollator, a locally hired scooter or taxi or hire car. Sometimes it was hard to do but it is not where you go, that does not matter, it is simply being able to do what you can, when you can, and enjoying your time doing it with someone you love.

Assistance

All airlines have an obligation to transport any disability aids, from walking sticks to rollators and large scooters free of charge. Do not let the fact that you use disability aids put you off travelling; just make sure that you can use what you are taking at your destination. Airlines also offer special assistance; you can arrange for a wheelchair to help you, from the time you arrive at the airport through to check-in. Speedy boarding is also helpful as it enables you to avoid crowds of people queueing at passport control and security. It also ensures that you board the plane first, so you can settle in your seat before everyone else gets on. When you land, you will always have to leave the plane last, but that does not matter as you will still reach baggage reclaim before everyone else, as you will probably be in a buggy.

Many airlines using UK airports have recently introduced special wheelchairs that enable a wheelchair user to transfer from their own chair to the aisle wheelchair and then to their seat. This can also be used during the flight to access the toilet easily. Be sure to book an aisle seat to make this process as easy as possible.

There have recently been some publicised instances where special assistance has not worked, for one reason or another; unfortunately, some disabled people have either lost wheelchairs or had difficulties on board the aircraft or in the terminal. By and large, we always found it worked for us; maybe we were lucky. Just ensure that you take full advantage of whatever help is available when you travel.

Before you book a holiday, it is worth checking to make sure that the resort is fully accessible, with lifts between floors and level access. Check the bathroom and shower facilities… Is the shower step-free, walk-in? Are there handrails? In other words, all the things you may be used to in your own home. Holiday companies should also be able to arrange whatever special assistance you need at the airport and on the plane. Your travel provider should be able to give you all this information and arrange whatever you need; if they are unable to do this, it means that they do not know the hotel and resort as well as they should, in providing you with what you need for an enjoyable and stress-free holiday.

If, for whatever reason, your holiday provider is unable to give you the information you need, contact the hotel direct. They should also be able to advise you what disabled access is like in their area.

If your provider is unable to help you, without you having to do the donkey work, maybe you should consider using another one. There are specialist holiday companies such as Limitless Travel and Enable Holidays, so it may be worth contacting them or researching similar companies.

Great Britain and Ireland

As well as going abroad, we also spent much time over the years travelling around Great Britain by car, not quite from Lands End to John O'Groats, but we visited and stayed in many places, including the West Country, the Lake District, Derbyshire, Yorkshire, West Midlands, the Scottish Borders, Wales and Dublin.

There is so much to see in this country, everywhere is generally accessible, including pavements and ramps for people with disabilities. Disability Discrimination Legislation mandates that service providers be legally obliged to make reasonable adjustments for individuals with disabilities. All the hotels we stayed in had suitable disabled access to entrances and facilities and suitable sized en suite showers, for example, as did the majority of B&Bs.

This may not always be the case, so always check the facilities of wherever you plan to stay, to make sure they are suitable for your needs.

Motorhomes

We always fancied the idea of going away in a motorhome, the freedom of travelling where and when you want, and to stop where you want, within reason, but always thought it would be too impractical for us. Lyn was now using her scooter all the time to go anywhere other than short walks with her walking stick so the year before the pandemic, just out of interest, we went to a local dealer to see what was available; The dealer showed us several; one, in particular, was very accessible for Lyn. She could get up the steps using the handrail and, once inside, everything was very easy to get around and use.

After we had looked over the vehicle, I asked the salesman, 'What about Lyn's scooter?'

He went to the side of the vehicle near the rear and opened a top-hung door, which revealed a storage space under one of the beds. It was more than big enough for a fold-down scooter like Lyn's and even had a charging point for the battery. I have recently checked online and there are now motorhomes with lifts, so fully accessible for wheelchair users. If you would like that type of holiday, it might just be possible.

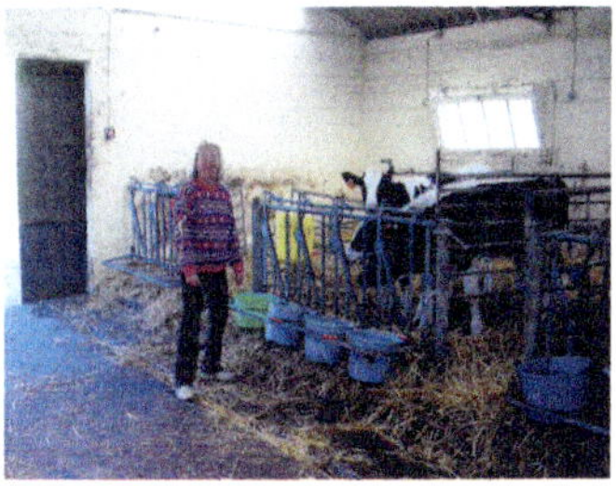

Vimoutiers. Lyn with the calves.

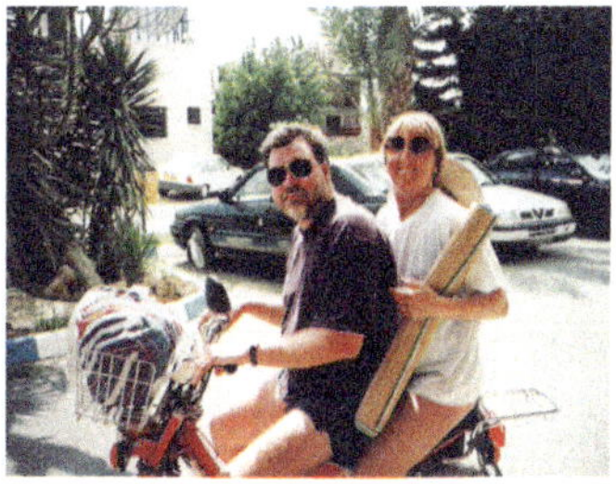

Cyprus, easy rider.

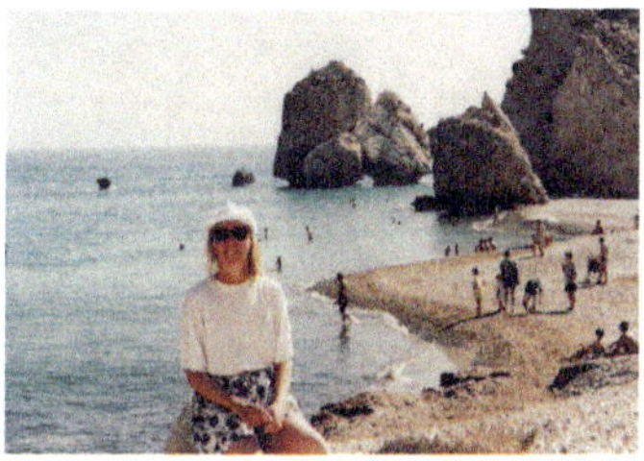

Cyprus, Aphrodite's Rock.

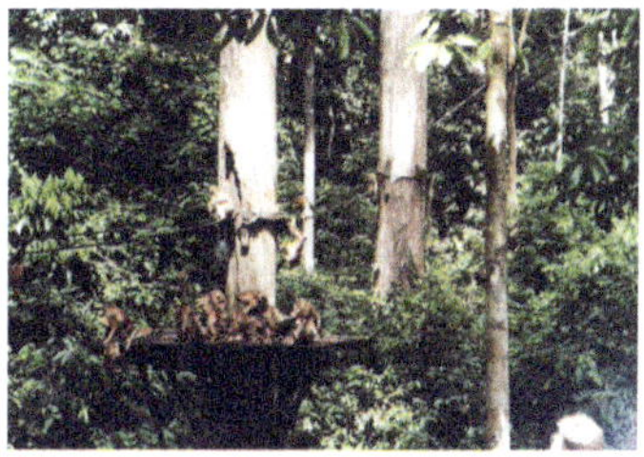

Borneo, Orangutan.

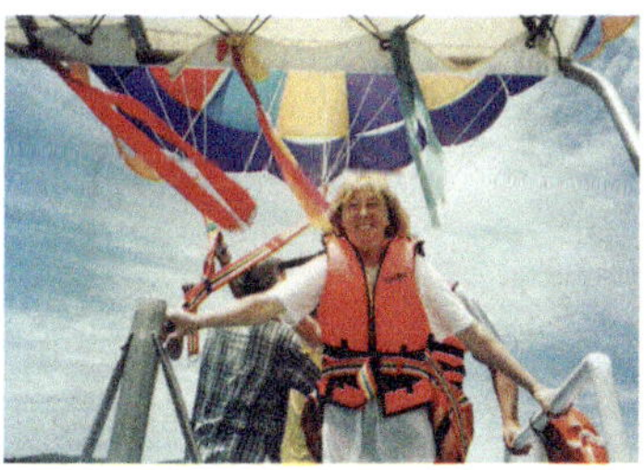

Borneo, ready to go parascending.

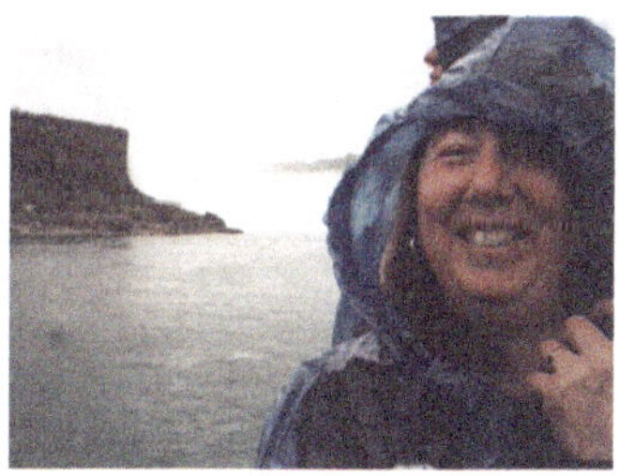

Canada, Niagara Falls, on the Maid of the Mist.

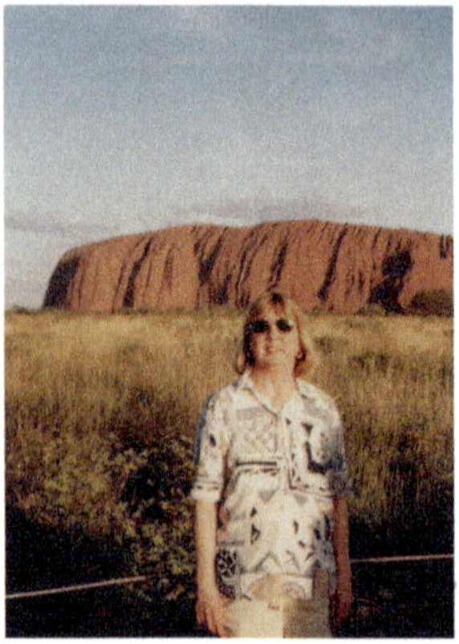

Australia, Uluru at dawn.

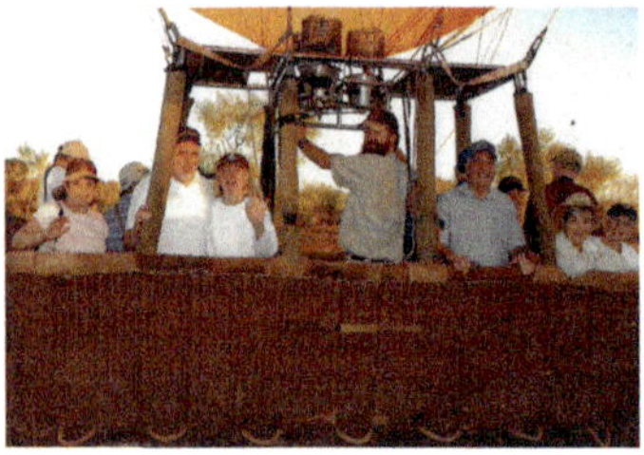

Australia, outback ballooning.

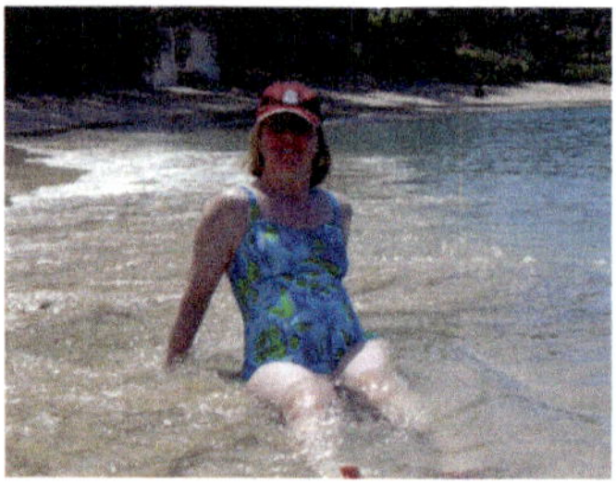

Barbados, relaxing.

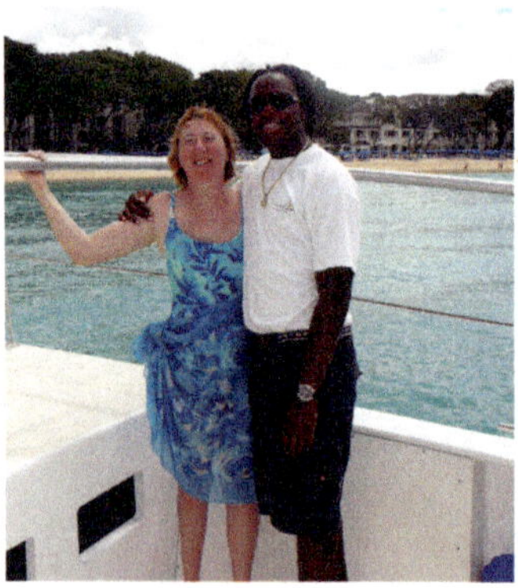

Barbados, Lyn with Captain Ahab.

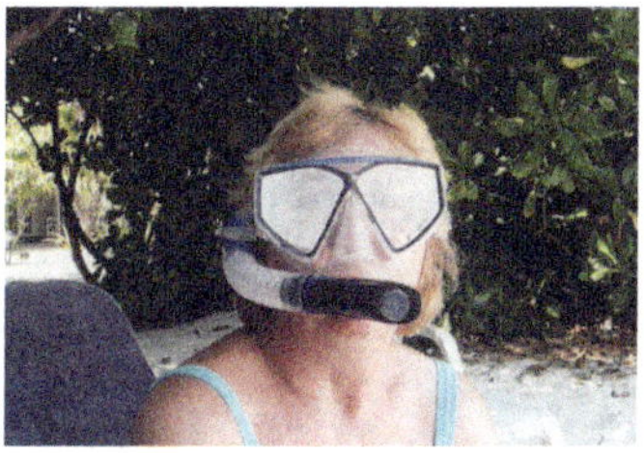

Maldives, getting ready to snorkel.

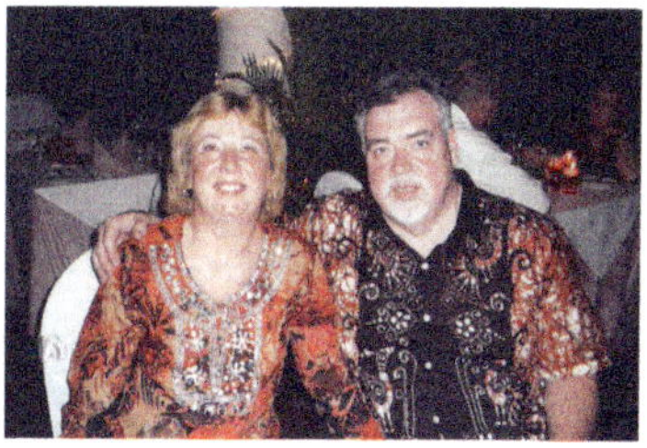

Sri Lanka, dressing up.

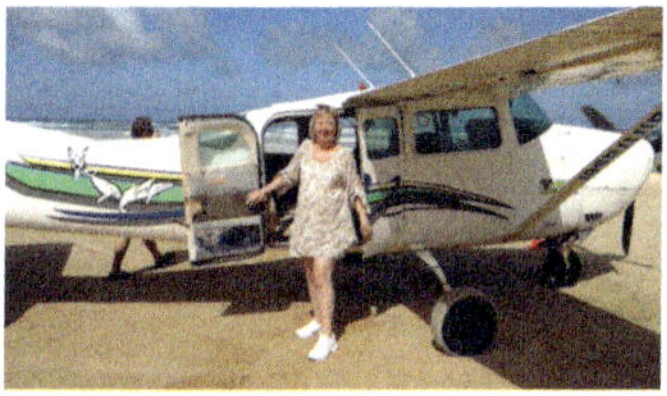

Australia, the plane on Fraser Island beach.

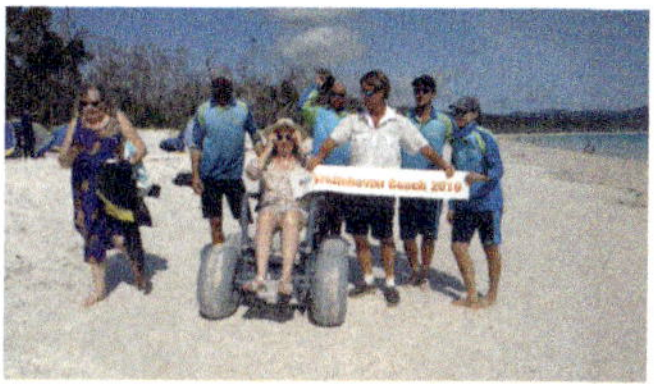

Australia, Whitsunday Island, balloon tyre wheelchair.

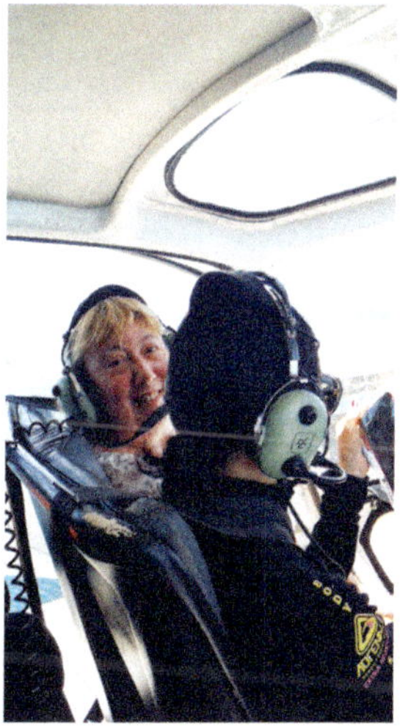

Australia, helicopter over Great Barrier Reef.

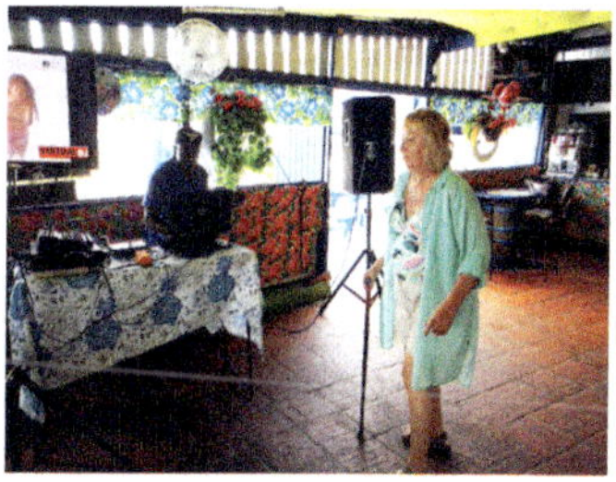

Barbados, Lyn dancing in her happy place.

27 Therapies

In Harrow, Lyn went to the MS therapy centre for some specific physiotherapy exercises, which she found very helpful; she tried to keep doing the exercises in the week after the sessions, as they did make a difference. It is vital to keep up these exercises at home, as you will benefit from them. Even doing them for half the time is better than not doing them at all. She would always meet people whom she knew, so there was plenty of social interaction as well, which is very important, especially if your disability means that your trips out might be limited.

The centre had a hyperbaric oxygen chamber, which many people with MS found beneficial; it is like deep-sea diving but on land in a chamber where you breathe pure oxygen. Lyn could never use this as she was claustrophobic; however, others with MS, who could use it, always said they felt better after a session.

Hyperbaric oxygen chamber (HBO)

The MS Society says:

> Some people with MS report benefits from using this type of treatment. But there's no scientific evidence that HBO therapy for multiple sclerosis works well. There are claims that this treatment may be helpful for managing your MS bladder.

> The NICE guideline for MS, which sets standards for treatment in the NHS in England, Wales and Northern Ireland, was updated in 2022. The updated guideline doesn't mention HBO therapy for treating MS in general. The only symptom it mentions is fatigue, where the new guideline doesn't recommend HBO therapy to treat it.
> You can find HBO treatment in most MS Therapy Centres. Usually hyperbaric oxygen doesn't cause serious side effects.

With MS, HBO is like many therapeutic treatments; sometimes there may be no medical evidence to support their positive effects on MS but, if some people feel the benefit of a particular treatment, it relieves symptoms, and has no adverse medical effects, then why not? If something makes you feel better, what is the harm in benefiting from it?

There are many MS therapy centres around the UK and it is worth contacting your local one as they offer plenty of help and advice. There is one in Exeter that Lyn went to for specialist physiotherapy exercises, where she also met many people over the years.

This is an extract from the Exeter website:

> The South West MS Therapy centre was established in 1982 as a self-funding charity initially to provide oxygen therapy, information and support for people with Multiple Sclerosis in the South West.
> From here the Centre developed to offer a number of therapies, not only for people with MS but also people

with other conditions. The Centre provides a welcoming and friendly environment, promoting independence and improving well-being and quality of life of our members and their families and carers.

We welcome members of all ages and are continually improving our facilities and treatments to suit a wide range of needs. Whether you are newly diagnosed or not, we strive to ensure you get access to all the information, support and therapies that can help you come to terms with and manage your symptoms.

When you enter the Centre you are greeted with a warm welcome by our team of friendly receptionists and other staff, members and our volunteers are always on hand to show you around.

There are comfy seats with a range of magazines and information leaflets to peruse, a plentiful selection of biscuits and cakes (optional!) to go with your freshly brewed tea or coffee from our newly fitted kitchen.

Alternatively, you can take a quieter break in our lounge a few steps away from reception with armchairs and a dining table.

Come and visit us for a no-obligation introductory tour, you'll be glad you did.

There are many centres across the country that are likely to share the same ethos and offer similar treatments. Lyn definitely benefitted from meeting other people. By talking to others, you gain more knowledge of how they deal with their symptoms, what exercises they do, and what treatments they are having. This all adds to your own knowledge of how to cope. If you do not try, you will never know what you might gain. I have only personal knowledge of the Harrow and Exeter Centres, details of which are in the Sources of Information section.

28 Driving

Lyn enjoyed driving, until she began to be wary of driving after dusk. This may be common with MS; it was not only Lyn, I know other people with MS who said they found it increasingly difficult to focus on the lights in front of them and gauge distances in the dark. Lyn never had a problem with distance vision and did not have an ophthalmic prescription for long-distance glasses. But she would become muddled, particularly on a motorway or main road, with tail lights directly in front of her and headlights coming towards her; on a curve in the road, all the lights would merge together.

She always preferred being a passenger but not only because of the lights; latterly, Lyn began to find driving generally quite tiring, even in the daytime.

Fatigue is a major part of MS and anything that makes fatigue worse is not good: concentration wavers, which leads to worrying about your driving, which leads to stress and that leads to other symptoms worsening.

It is not a question of not driving, rather a question of the person with MS knowing when to stop—and for the carer to recognise it as well. But in 1998, Lyn wanted to prove to herself that she could drive long distances on her own. She and her friend, Val, drove to Folkestone, boarded the Eurotunnel train to Calais and then drove down to Vimoutiers in Normandy to stay with our friends, Chrissie and Tim, for a few days. Lyn drove Val to the places we had visited and enjoyed on our many previous visits. A few days later, she drove back home; they were both in one piece and had enjoyed the drive to and around Normandy and their time spent with Chrissie and Tim. Val drove them back from Folkestone to Harrow.

Lyn drove about 900 miles on that trip and thoroughly enjoyed it and I was more worried about her driving round the M25 than driving in France; although it has many more registered cars than the UK, France is a much larger country so roads seem quieter. Lyn had proved to herself that she could do it. Sometimes that is enough.

After we moved to Somerset, Lyn drove to larger local towns about 40 miles away and was fine, although she liked company when driving. Occasionally, she drove back to Harrow Weald to see her stepmother, and to Leighton Buzzard or Bristol to see our daughters, with me as passenger; sometimes if I were working, I would come back by train and she would stay on for a few days and then drive back on her own. For me, the worst part of her drive home was worrying about the M4 / M5 interchange, which can take many drivers by surprise, but she managed it.

Lyn continued to drive, but she was very much a fair-weather daytime driver; as her MS progressed, she felt less confident in driving any distance and would prefer to be a passenger. She had to drive me to hospital and visit me a couple of times, not long after we had moved, but she would always prefer some company when she drove, as it gave her more confidence.

Everyone is different and the driving ability of anyone with MS can obviously vary. What you must do is to advise the DVLA if you have been diagnosed with MS.

This means that you have to re-apply for a new licence every three years, and your GP has to confirm your fitness to drive. You should also notify your insurer, otherwise, in the event of an accident you will not be covered. This does not mean that you cannot drive; it merely means that you have taken the necessary steps to allow you to continue to drive and to enjoy driving for as long as you can, and to feel safe doing so.

29 The things you do

Dancing

If there was one thing Lyn loved it was dancing. In her early teens, she went to the Guy Hayward School of Dancing in Harrow. She learned the standard ballroom dances, including the waltz and quickstep and, although other interests took over, she still liked to dance. We did not go to many formal dances, where she could have shown me her moves, but we did go to a few discos.

Lyn also loved the annual dinner dance that the firm I worked for held, in the late 1970s and early 1980s, at top London hotels, like the Inn on the Park or the Dorchester She enjoyed the chance to dress up for the evening in a posh frock, the ambience, the friends, the drinks and the dancing…she loved it all.

As Lyn's MS progressed, the dancing became more of a slow rhythmic movement on the spot, which was absolutely fine; she still enjoyed it, as well as listening to the music.

It will be no surprise that one of her favourite TV shows was *Strictly Come Dancing*, it was almost a ritual in our home. On a Saturday evening, we would sit in the living room, with an easy supper on a tray, and settle down to watch. I grew to like it too; the skill of those dancers was quite something.

College courses

Lyn was interested in many different things and subjects

and, over the years, she managed to do so much. In 1999, when our youngest daughter, Kelly, was studying A-levels at college, Lyn decided she wanted to study A-level Geography. She had passed Geography O-level at school but never had the chance to go on to A-levels at a further education college. She went along to Stanmore College once a week and the course included completing a study of a local amenity and analysing how much the local community used it.

Lyn chose a local area of common ground called Bentley Priory, which was part of the Harrow Weald Common public open space. We had walked there with the girls since we moved to Harrow Weald; it was not just a common space, it also had an enclosure with different types of deer, which we used to feed. Part of the study involved collating information on frequency of use by the public and establish their experience and enjoyment, for example. I would go along with her for company and, as she was starting to have dexterity issues, help her record the information, while she asked the questions.

Lyn completed the course, took the final exam, and Kelly went with her to pick up her result. She came out of the college with an envelope and said, excitedly, 'I got a U. What does that mean?'

'It means ungraded, Mum.'

'Oh well, at least I did it.'

That typified Lyn's approach to life; it does not matter if you do not pass with flying colours, as long as you tried and enjoyed it.

Although Lyn tired easily, she always knew that

mornings were her best time to do anything. She did quite a few adult courses at Harrow Weald College; painting and drawing was one she enjoyed but calligraphy was one of her favourites. Dexterity problems made it quite difficult for her but she still managed to complete the course and I still have all her work.

Lyn also took a pottery course, making hand-moulded pots and vases and other objects like pineapples; she managed to throw bowls on the potter's wheel. I still have all these as well.

Once, she came home and said, 'We've got a live model next week; I don't know what we'll be doing.' When she arrived home after the following week's class, she said that the live model had been a man. When the students arrived, he was already sitting completely naked on a chair in Rodin's *Thinker* pose. They had to make a hand-moulded model of him in all his glory...She opened the box she had bought the clay model home in, as she had to make any finishing touches at home before returning a week later to put him in the oven to fire before glazing.

On the morning that Lyn was taking him back to college, I must have had the devil in me; while she was getting ready, I could not resist taking a spare piece of clay and creating a perfectly formed but huge erect penis and moulding it into place over the rather flaccid member she had created. Lyn came into the kitchen, took one look, put both hands up to her mouth, laughed and said, 'Oh my God, what have you done? I can't take him like that—what will they think?'

'Creative interpretation,' I said, innocently.

Sadly, he had to lose his aroused manhood for the sake

of public decency. Pity, really. It was a very good model and I have kept the finished piece.

Flying

Lyn had always wanted to experience flying a small plane so, in 1997, I bought her a trial lesson at Elstree Aerodrome. She found it a little difficult to get into the cockpit but managed it with some help and flew for about thirty minutes. The pilot took her on a good flight over north west London and the surrounding countryside and she loved it, not least the opportunity, mid-air, to take the controls before the pilot landed.

Lyn had an amazing day.

Water skiing

In 2005, Lyn learned that it was possible to try water skiing. A group of people with a varying disabilities met at an old sand quarry, off the M4 near Heathrow Airport; it had been flooded to form a lake and turned into a water sports centre. Lyn got into a dry suit with my help—there was a vague resemblance to a Michelin man—and then went water skiing, supported on either side by two rather hunky men. They all sat on the deck with their feet on skis dangling over the side, holding onto a long bar fixed to the rope attached to the boat. The boat started up and they were off, heading around the lake a few times before returning. Lyn's face was a picture; she had thoroughly enjoyed the experience. There were a couple of others from the local MS branch who also had a go.

About twenty people with disabilities, including single and double, arm and leg amputees, and one visually impaired man, were taking part that day. There were different types of skis, such as mono skis, and a canoe-type ski that allowed anyone with a disability to experience water skiing.

If you want to try something new or different, there is always a way to achieve it and there are now more places than ever that offer all-inclusive activities.

Knitting

Shortly after the pandemic ended, Lyn wanted to teach our granddaughter, Bethany, to knit, but had forgotten some of the simple techniques. I asked our friend, Shuna, who is involved in a local knitting group, if she could go over the basics with Lyn. Shuna was more than happy to help and Lyn spent an afternoon, refreshing her skills, which she was then able to show Bethany a week later. It was not easy with her dexterity issues but she persevered.

Family

Family meant everything to both of us and over the years we spent as much time as possible with Sarah and Steve, Kelly and Keith, and grandchildren, Matt, Will, Hayden and Bethany. This was very precious time and always enjoyable.

After we moved to Dulverton, they often came to stay for longer, which was good for everyone. All the grandchildren helped with the garden and other things, and we visited many different places. But mostly they enjoyed spending as many hours as possible in the swimming pool.

Celebrations

Lyn and I always celebrated our birthdays and wedding anniversaries. We would usually have lunch somewhere or a day out, with lunch or at least coffee and cake. Sarah and Kelly knew that these celebrations meant a lot to Lyn and, on a couple of memorable occasions, the girls treated us to something special.

We went for lunch one Mother's Day at a pleasant local hotel, Lyn loved the meal but, when the desserts arrived, hers was a bowl of small cubes of jelly, fruit, blobs of custard and cream, with a sauce artistically drizzled over it. She looked aghast at the offering and asked the waiter, 'What's this?'

'It's deconstructed trifle, madam.' Lyn had misread the menu…

'Just get me a real one, please.'

Lyn enjoyed her food. She even stole things from my plate if I were not looking, especially if it was a pudding she liked. But I was not the only victim…She was an opportunist; grandson, Will, would not sit next to her—in case she stole *his* food.

Murder mystery

In the early 2000s, they booked a murder mystery trip on a train from Waterloo to Brighton. It was set in the 1930s and the carriages were classic 1930s style, there were flowers on the tables, and the train staff were suitably dressed too. We had a champagne breakfast on the train and met the cast members; then it was on to Brighton and lunch in the Royal Pavilion, where the murder took place. On the return journey, we had to guess the identity of the murderer…we won and received an Agatha Christie novel as a prize.

40th anniversary

When we opened our many cards that morning, there was one from the girls. The only writing inside was a postcode and a note that said, 'Pack for two nights and days.' Later that morning we followed the satnav to a hotel, where a bottle of bubbly and a bowl of fruit awaited us. We had two wonderful nights and days in a fine country house hotel with its own grounds.

Days out

We frequently took off for the day, sometimes knowing where we were going, mostly not. We often went to Lyme Regis, a favourite place, to Lynton and Lynmouth, or to another of the places we had come to know. It never took much to please Lyn; she had very simple tastes and was quite happy just spending time together, with me walking next to her on her scooter, visiting art galleries and potteries, or having lunch at a favourite pub or restaurant—simple pleasures.

Dressing up

We used to hold an occasional New Year's Eve party and insisted that everyone dressed up. If someone had nothing to wear, there were always a couple of black bin liners full of bits and pieces, ours and the girls', so there was no excuse.

The last time that Lyn and I dressed up was at a fancy

dress party in the early 2000s, hosted by John, the drummer of the band I played with. I went as Freddie Mercury, dyed my moustache and beard black, and put on tight black leggings and a yellow sleeveless vest. Lyn went as Tina Turner; we managed to get a wig from the local market, she had a suitable dress and some high-heeled shoes that she had been unable able to wear for some time. We were all set to go and, even given Lyn's difficulty with walking and the challenging high-heels, she pulled off Tina Turner's stage walk perfectly. The costumes went down really well and it was a great party. Lyn took off those shoes as soon as she could…

After being diagnosed with MS, Lyn was always willing to try different things and she achieved so much. Although MS restricted what she could do physically, she believed that it was not about what you do but, rather, about not letting your disability rule your life.

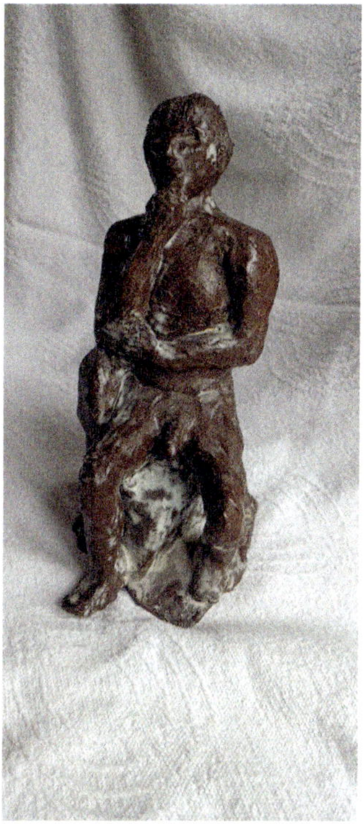

Pottery course, thinking man.

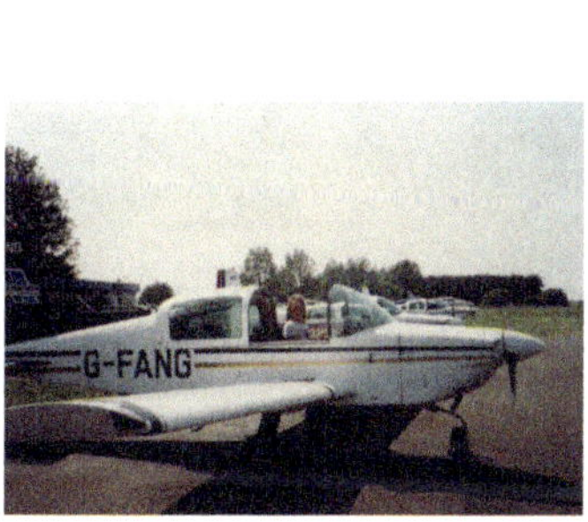

Lyn ready for her flying lesson.

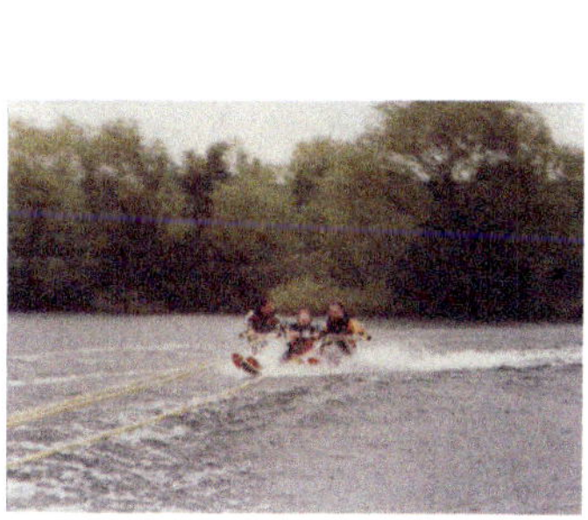

Lyn water skiing.

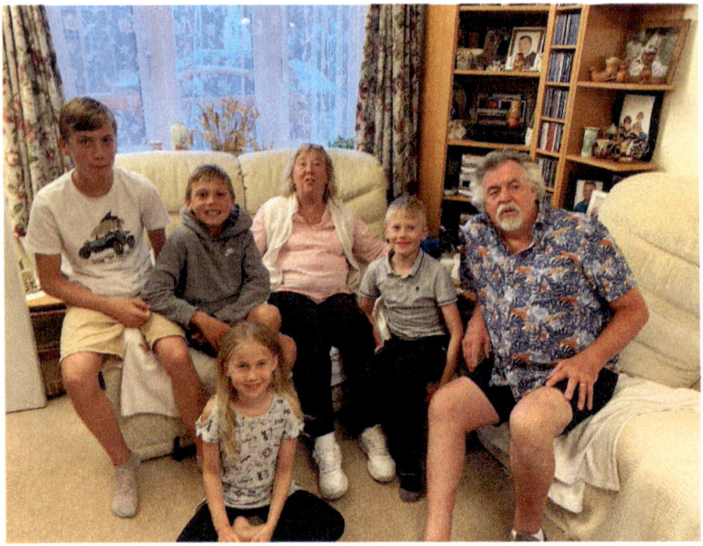

With the grandchildren, 2021.

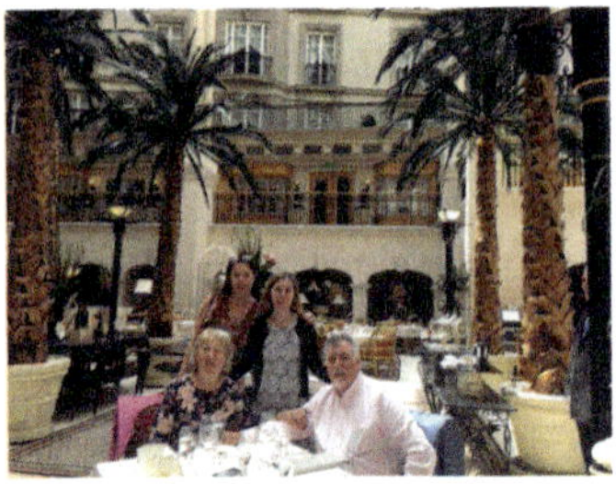

Lunch with our girls.

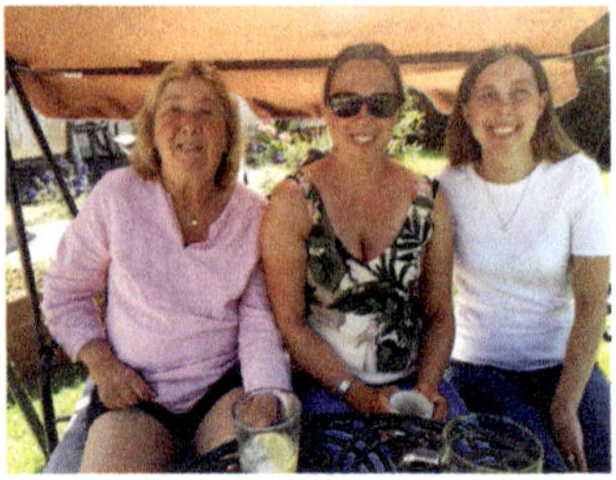

Chilling on a swing.

30 Music, gigs and theatre, continued

After moving, our interest in music remained the same; the radio or CD player was always on, providing background music during the day. One Christmas, Kelly bought us an Alexa, which I still use as there is such an incredible amount of music available on demand.

In more recent years, we saw Peter Frampton at Bristol O2 and also KT Tunstall, The Pretenders and Simple Minds in an open air gig at Taunton Racecourse, where there was a section set aside for disabled people with wheelchairs or scooters, right in front of the stage; an ideal place to sit and watch. Lyn was convinced that Jim Kerr was actually singing to her.

At the Peter Frampton gig, we were in the disabled seating area, which had a great view of the stage, marred only by a couple in the main seating in front of us. The man repeatedly made loud comments on Peter talking about each song, and was generally being a pain. Asking him to lower his voice but he became stroppy. However, one of the security team had a word with him and he stopped. After the interval, the couple did not return. The burly security man approached us and said, 'The gentleman won't be coming back to annoy you sir, madam; he decided to leave of his own accord,' He was turfed out then…

The last time we saw *Les Misérables* was in 2015, at the Queen's Theatre (now the Sondheim Theatre), in London's Shaftesbury Avenue. As usual, we had arranged for disabled access; a host met us in the foyer and escorted us via a side entrance in Wardour Street to our seats, which were on the same level. He took our coats, came back at the interval to help with drinks, and escorted us out at the end. I would think that same help and attentiveness is still available and at most, if not all, theatres.

It is always worth checking a venue's disabled facilities, either via its website or by telephoning; you will always find staff helpful.

A few years after we moved to Dulverton, our friends, Pam and Steve, had created an open-air theatre in their extensive garden. The ground's shape lent itself to carving a three-tier amphitheatre, which was then grassed over. It provided a wonderful outdoor theatre environment, which was easily accessible for Lyn on her scooter, and we attended several enjoyable productions.

At one production that we went to a few years ago, with Kelly, Keith, Hayden and Bethany, Lyn was sitting on her scooter, I was on a picnic chair, and the others were on blankets. I was quite happy until, without warning, my chair collapsed under me; my arms and legs went upwards, my pint of beer disappeared behind me, and I ended up like a tortoise on its back, all four limbs waving in the air. Predictably, this caused much mirth and laughter from all around me, including the players, who were quite happy to watch while I struggled to right myself, until some kind soul eventually took pity on me and helped me up. The play resumed; I sat on the grass and someone bought me a beer.

I have continued to go to gigs either with friends, Sarah, or grandson, Matt, and I will be taking my other grandchildren as they get older.

31 Lynisms

Lyn would always get a bit mixed up with certain names and sayings, whether malapropisms are a common thing for people with MS, I do not know; maybe it was just Lyn…

Oots and boos — boots and shoes
Botticellis — Andrea Bocelli, tenor
Dick Raspberry — Rick Astley, singer
Tuilangies — Manu Tuilagi, rugby player
Jomi Lomi — Jonah Lomu, New Zealand rugby player
Nesty Dormouse — Nessun' Dorma
Julio needs glasses — Julio Iglesias
Ceylon John — Céline Dion
Muckin' fuddle — you can work that one out

and many more.

32 Treatments

There are many different ways to manage MS, depending on the type and symptoms; these include drug treatments, DMT's, disease modifying therapies, exercise, diet and other lifestyle changes.

The MS Society produces a booklet on *Treatments and Therapies,* this is an extract from their website:

> It's best to get advice on your multiple sclerosis treatment with a specialist, like a neurologist. An MS nurse can discuss treatment for MS generally, but only an MS specialist can advise you and prescribe treatment. The types of treatments and therapies that may be beneficial for you will depend on your type of MS and your symptoms. Some therapies and treatments for MS treat the symptoms. For instance, you might need physiotherapy to help you improve your strength and mobility. Others, such as disease moderating therapies (DMTs) and haematopoietic stem cell transplantation (HSCT) manage MS itself.
>
> There are around twenty DMTs licensed to treat relapsing and some forms of progressive MS. Taking one can mean you get fewer, and less serious, relapses. They can also slow down how fast your MS gets worse.
>
> Lots of people with MS find it useful to actively manage their health in other ways, like through diet, exercise or giving up smoking.

Disease modifying treatment (DMT) decision tool

There's a wide range of DMTs for MS available on the NHS. Each has a different combination of benefits and risks.

Use our tool to explore your DMT options and prepare for conversations with health.

Not every DMT is available to everyone. And the tool can't tell you which you qualify to get on the NHS. Your neurologist can tell you that after they have examined you and seen your MRI scans.

If you are using this tool on behalf of someone with MS, answer the questions as if you are that person.

Who's this tool for?

You can use this tool if you live in the UK, Channel Islands or Isle of Man and have:

relapsing remitting MS

some types of primary or secondary progressive MS.

If you have progressive MS, it must be active MS to use this tool. 'Active' means your MRI scans show signs of recent inflammation. You might also still get relapses. If your progressive MS isn't active, unfortunately there are no DMTs available at the moment. You also won't qualify for a DMT if you use a wheelchair all the time.

Some people might not qualify for a DMT. If so, other treatments and lifestyle changes can help with your MS symptoms. Trials of new drugs for progressive MS are underway. Find out more about the trials taking us closer to treatments for everyone.

How long does the tool take? Check this online on the MS

> Society website.
> You can finish it in about 15 to 20 minutes. Use it as many times as you like. It will suggest more DMTs if you give answers with fewer restrictions.

While many treatments for different types of MS were developed over the years, at the time Lyn was diagnosed—and up until 2022—there were no specific drug treatments for primary progressive MS. There was always information about much of the research in the UK and US in many publications. There is now a chance that a treatment for primary progressive MS is on the horizon. As noted above, there are some treatments for progressive MS but it must be active. This is an extract from the MS Society website about the current trials for progressive MS:

> Octopus is being led by Professor Jeremy Chataway. Jeremy says, "The multi-arm, multi-stage approach to trialing emerging medications has been utterly transformative in other conditions. So I'm thrilled we're now able to apply it to progressive MS. Ultimately, Octopus will lead to more treatments for progression becoming available to people living with MS sooner.
> "Getting to this stage has been an incredible joint effort of people up and down the country. The other large trial I am Chief Investigator for, MS-STAT2, has shown we can run large-scale, nationwide trials for progressive MS. Now we're taking it to the next level as we start a new journey to develop treatments for progressive MS. I know our amazing community of people is poised to help us make it to the top, so we can find the answers we so desperately

need."

Professor Max Parmar, Director of the Medical Research Council Clinical Trials Unit at UCL, is co-leading Octopus with Jeremy. He's a trial design expert who helped change how men with prostate cancer around the world are treated.

Dr Emma Gray, our Assistant Director of Research, says "Launching the world's first multi-arm, multi-stage trial for MS has long been an ambition of ours. And opening the doors to Octopus is a momentous milestone. More than 130,000 people live with MS in the UK. And there are tens of thousands with progressive forms who have nothing to stop their MS getting worse. By tapping into the potential of approved drugs, which may have the potential to protect nerves, we can develop new treatments for MS faster.

"This is a major moment for MS research – Octopus has the potential to change the clinical trials landscape around the world. It's thanks to all the wonderful participants that trials, like Octopus, can happen. We won't stop until we have treatments that transform the lives of everyone with MS."

Hopefully, this research and others around the world will result in a drug treatment that will benefit everybody with primary progressive MS.

33 Life with MS—later years

Lyn's MS symptoms became progressively worse in the years since her original diagnosis. Early on, the first noticeable symptoms were her balance getting worse and some spasticity in her legs, which made walking awkward. Next, she had more difficulty walking and mobilising generally; she progressed from using my arm every day, to a walking stick or frame all the time, and then a rollator. Her bladder started to be affected; the most noticeable symptom was 'Mrs Frequently'—she needed to know that there was a toilet available, wherever we went. This was nothing new but had become worse.

Lyn's walking worsened, slowly but perceptibly; we saw physiotherapists regularly at the MS therapy centre in Harrow, then Exeter and, latterly, a specialist physiotherapist in Taunton, to go over exercises aimed at maintaining muscle tone in her legs. Doing exercises with a physiotherapist is relatively easy, as you get into a routine; carrying them on at home is not so easy as you need motivation. Lyn did try to do these at home and I helped her to do them, physically and by nagging her to keep doing them.

I have been as bad as anyone else in keeping up with physiotherapy after surgery; it is not easy. But it is so important to keep up the exercises that a physiotherapist suggests, as it will help you to maintain that muscle tone. It also helps to have someone who can encourage you.

As mentioned previously, that old adage, 'Use it or lose

it,' is true. If you do not walk or exercise regularly, even a little, you will lose muscle tone and strength and, the older you become, the harder it is to restore. That is why it is important to use organisations like the MS therapy centres, who can provide expert advice on which types of exercise are best for you, your type of MS, and your symptoms.

Even though Lyn continued with these exercises, her MS did, inevitably and slowly, progress; by the mid-2000s, she was using her rollator almost all the time to help get around. In 2008-9, Lyn started using the scooter when she went anywhere, such as Kew Gardens, that would have involved walking any distance. It enabled her to get around more easily, keep up with everyone else, and not feel she was holding anyone up.

Most gardens and houses open to the public have accessible routes for either ambulant disabled people needing a more even or flatter surface, or for those with rollators, wheelchairs or scooters. Most also have wheelchairs and scooters freely available or for hire by anyone with a disability. Always telephone or check online in advance to check what help is available and what equipment they have, as you may need to book before you visit.

Once we had moved and settled in to our new home, we made contact with the Exeter branch of the MS Society and found out that there was a local support group in Tiverton, so Lyn contacted them and we started going to their monthly lunch meetings. It was another group of delightful people, all in a similar situation to so many others with MS; some, like Lyn, had primary progressive MS and others were not so good. Nevertheless, there was that same spirit and camaraderie that you find in a group of people with a disease in common.

One day, we were having a coffee at the Copper Kettle in Dulverton, when a couple we had not seen before walked in and sat at the table next to us. We struck up a conversation, as we normally did… The lady had gone to use the toilet and, when she came back, Lyn said, 'Don't mind me asking but have you got MS?'

'Yes, I've got primary progressive.'

'I thought I recognised the gait.'

That started another friendship; Lyn told them about the Tiverton support group and they joined as well.

After a couple of years living in Dulverton, Lyn predictably wanted to do something to help raise funds for the local group; one of the things she organised was a 'Cake Break', a staple MS Society fundraiser. This involved local people in baking large or small cakes and selling them on a particular day; the support at that first event was very encouraging. Hanover Court, a local housing rental property that provides apartments with extra care for elderly people, allowed us to use their communal lounge as a venue. Their catering staff also provided cakes, as well as coffee and tea. These were all sold in portions on the day and all the money raised was split between the local MS support group and the national MS Society; plenty of funds were raised this way, over the years.

After we had moved to Dulverton, we tried to get some exercise equipment that Lyn could use easily. We wanted a treadmill similar to the one that she had been able to use easily at the Mike Heaffey Centre. The difficulty she had now, as her MS had developed, was using the type at the gym—as soon as you pressed the button, it started at a certain pace; slow as it was, it would still take her by surprise and would put her off balance. So we bought a self-propelled version, rather than a powered treadmill; you stepped onto it and it moved when you moved. Good? No, sadly; it was so well set up that by putting just one foot on the treadmill, the belt started moving immediately, sending you off balance. There was no way, she could get both feet on before it started moving. We managed to sell that one locally. Lesson learned; always try out something like that in a shop before buying online.

We also bought a rowing machine; although Lyn tried it and could use it on a low resistance setting, the problem was getting on, as it meant getting down on her knees, swinging her bottom sideways, sitting on the seat, and then swinging her legs over the frame to get her feet onto the pedals. Too many things to think about and co-ordinate, if you have MS. There are now several types of rowing machines for disabled people, some with higher seats than normal, some that can be used from a wheelchair. Some gyms and leisure centres have them, but not all; check locally to see what is available to suit you.

I bought an exercise bike, mainly for me, which I was quite happy using. Lyn also tried it but she could not get onto the saddle, even at the lowest height. We visited a shop that sold various types of exercise equipment and found an exercise bike that Lyn could use—a recumbent cycle, which had a lower seat than the other exercise bike. You sit in a reclining position; your back is fully supported and your legs are on the pedals straight ahead of you. Lyn found this much easier and used it while she could. I could not use it as your feet splay outwards in that position and, due to the previous operations on my feet, my ankle bones always hit the pedal crank.

For about five years up until the start of the pandemic, Lyn went to an exercise class in Dulverton; it was run by Nicola, who led Zumba classes, including a less strenuous class for older people, who could not move that quickly or easily. The class members were behind chairs, for support when needed or for seated exercise. Lyn enjoyed the classes, there were plenty of movements that worked various muscle groups to music. Everyone knew each other, so there was a good deal of banter too.

This was all good; exercise and meeting people are both important. Even if you are unable to do much exercise, you will probably find a class that works for you and gives you a chance to socialise. Try your local MS Society branch, disability groups or the local town website.

Lyn also went to Isis Wellbeing and Skin Care in Dulverton, which provided massage therapies and beauty treatments, such as Calgel nails. Zoe, the massage therapist was very skilled and also did therapeutic massage; Lyn always felt better for a thorough back and neck massage. Gina did the nail treatments, which Lyn liked to have every few months; she always tried to look her best. Having a conversation at the same time was therapeutic, as well. Lyn also wanted her hair to look as good and went to Emma at Hows the Hair, every four weeks or so for a wash, cut and blow-dry and, of course, chatting over coffee.

These were all therapies that made Lyn feel good about herself, which is very important for anyone.

Everyone who knew Lyn said that she was always

smiling and had a kind word for everyone. Even when things were at their worst, she still had an indomitable spirit and would not give in easily. That was Lyn's way of dealing with things; if she were suffering inside, she never let it show. There was always that smile and being happy to talk to people. Showing anger about your circumstances all the time, can be pretty wearing and self-destructive and will dissuade people from communicating with you.

In 2018, Lyn was referred to a specialist neuro-physiotherapy unit, to see if her walking and pain relief could be improved. She tried different exercises over a few months. It was then suggested that she try using a TENS machine.

The MS Society website has this description:

> Transcutaneous electrical nerve stimulation (TENS) involves using a mild, low voltage electric current to treat pain. It can be used to treat some types of pain in multiple sclerosis, such as:
>
> Burning, tingling or shooting pains where there is no obvious reason
> Back pain - often caused by reduced mobility or poor posture;
> Spasticity and painful leg spasms, where anti-spasmodic medications are not tolerated.

TENS can reduce pain in the short-term but does not get rid of the pain or the underlying problem permanently. Often TENS is something that needs to be used on a long-term basis, but it can improve quality of life and reduce the need to take pain medications for:

nerve pain (neuropathic pain) which is caused by damage to the nerves in the brain and spinal cord. This includes altered sensations such as pins and needles, numbness, crawling or burning feelings. Examples of nerve pain include painful sensations in the side of the face, called trigeminal neuralgia, and a tight feeling, often around the chest, called the MS hug. Pain in the limbs is very common.

Musculoskeletal (nociceptive) pain which is caused by damage to muscles, tendons, ligaments and soft tissue, for example neck or back pain caused by changes in posture or sitting for very long periods.

We went to the physiotherapy unit at Cotford St Luke to try the TENS machine. It consists of a control unit connected to electrodes that are placed wherever necessary to provide the stimulation, while the intensity is adjusted via the control unit. Lyn tried it at various intensities and it did reduce the pain and helped overcome the spasticity in her right leg, but she felt that the sensations of the electrical impulses were quite uncomfortable. As well as helping the spasticity, it allowed her to move her right leg without it dragging.

One thing Lyn was worried about was going home with the unit and telling the grandchildren how it worked. They might have had great fun turning up the dial and watching Nanny walk around the room at increasing speeds, like Wallace in *The Wrong Trousers.*

The TENS machine may suit some people with MS but

it might not be for everyone. However, it is always worth trying these things, as they may well work for you.

Lyn always had a positive attitude and was willing to find out about any potential cures; although there were none available for primary progressive MS, there was always talk of drug trials and continuing research. After moving to Dulverton in 2010, Lyn attended the Royal Devon and Exeter Hospital Neurology Department. Her consultant was Dr Tim Harrower, who is now an associate professor at the University of Exeter Medical School, another delightful man, in whom Lyn had much faith. He was always willing to spend time talking with her about any concerns or increasing symptoms she had, or changing medications if needed.

Lyn told Dr Harrower to put her name down for any drug trials he was aware of, but sadly her age was against her; the trials wanted younger people with MS who, realistically, were likely to feel any benefits over a longer period. That did not stop her, however, as she desperately wanted to take part in research. One day, she was discussing this with her specialist nurse, Louise, at Tiverton and District Hospital. Louise was very empathetic and, over the years, had developed an excellent relationship with Lyn. She told Lyn about a Plymouth University trial that would provide research data on certain aspects of MS. Lyn's tenacity came to the fore again and she wasted no time in volunteering for the trial, more of which later.

34 Incontinence

This is rarely an easy thing for anyone to talk about. Incontinence is one of those MS symptoms that most people with MS can suffer with, as the bladder is a muscle that can be affected like so many others. I am not exactly sure when it started with Lyn; it crept up on us, like other symptoms. The first thing I noticed was that, whenever we went anywhere, she would always need to go for a pee, so would always ask where we were going and where the toilets were.

After a few years, we had to carefully plan any car journeys to make sure we had stopping points. It was not until about 2013 that Lyn's incontinence started to become worse, to the point that she needed some protection all the time. She started using incontinence pants; initially they were not that bulky, as some are quite thin, more female, types that could be used when she was at home, for example. Over time, Lyn needed the thicker types for greater protection, which gave her more confidence when we were out.

There are also several types of men's incontinence pants, available in pharmacies, supermarkets, or in bulk online. Lyn always preferred to buy online as it was more convenient and less embarrassing than walking around the supermarket with them in the trolley.

It reached the stage when Lyn would sometimes go through three to four pairs of incontinence pants in twenty-four hours; she might wake in the middle of the night, feeling the need to change and, occasionally, she would also wet the bed, which meant a sheet change as well. I had to help Lyn to change all the time due to her mobility and dexterity issues and, at nights, she would invariably be very tired; this made it even more difficult for me, as what she could do to help was limited. This continual change of pants and cleaning up did have an effect on our more intimate life, but you have to work your way through these things, difficult as they may be.

On our last holiday, in February 2020, it reached the point that we had one small suitcase containing nothing but incontinence pants, as we did not know if we could buy them abroad. You might have to factor that into your luggage allowance…

In 2017, Sarah took Lyn for a long weekend trip to Majorca, for some mother-daughter time; Sarah found the help that Lyn needed challenging, to say the least, but she did all she could to make her mum's trip as enjoyable as possible, and Lyn really enjoyed the trip.

Lyn was never doubly incontinent; in fact, quite the reverse, as her bowels were very sluggish. This is common with MS as the bowels are another group of muscles that can be affected and not work properly. For about ten years, it was normal for Lyn to sometimes go three to five days without having a poo. She did not feel much discomfort, it was simply the amount of time her system took to work things through.

Constipation can be caused or aggravated by several factors: lack of exercise, not drinking enough water, not enough fruit and vegetables, some medications, and even ageing.

Our diet was pretty good, fish, chicken and fruit and vegetables, not much red meat, and plenty of water. Lyn's ability to exercise was limited but she did what she could; it was simply her constitution. If she was very uncomfortable and constipated, had been unable to go for some time but felt she needed to go, some massaging with oil and gentle pressing over her tummy for a while helped things to move along a little.

The only downside to having little control over your bowels is that you might need to go at any time. There was often no warning so it was just as well that Lyn always wore the incontinence pants; they prevented many a potentially embarrassing moment. If that happened while we were driving, I had to find somewhere to deal with the incident and help Lyn clean up. Whenever we went out, even on a short trip, we always made sure we had spare pants, as well as plenty of wet wipes and tissues and a change of clothes, as we never knew when she might need them. These may sound like extreme measures, but you have to anticipate these things and allow for them whenever you travel anywhere; it can save much embarrassment and heartache.

In 2021, I started suffering temporarily with incontinence and was peeing intermittently. Little did I know that this was a precursor to retention caused by a benign enlarged prostate, so I now had first-hand experience and appreciated what Lyn was going through with those pants as I had to use them too.

Here is some advice from the MS Society website:

Carry our free 'I need some help' card. It explains you have MS and urgently need the toilet.

Get it by calling 0300 500 8084 or email supportercare@mssociety.org.uk.

Find a public toilet at Toilet Map or download one of the public toilet apps.

Join the National (RADAR) Key Scheme. For a few pounds you get a key that lets you into over 9,000 locked accessible toilets in the UK.

If you need a public toilet bigger than standard accessible ones, or you need a hoist, check out Changing Places.

Contact your council to see if there's a Community Toilets Scheme locally. It lets you use toilets in shops, restaurants and pubs without paying.

35 Gardening

Lyn always loved flowers and liked gardening but, as her symptoms progressed, her ability to help with the gardening gradually decreased. In Harrow Weald, we had quite a small garden—about 16 by 12 metres—which was typical for a 1930s semi-detached house. We grew mainly shrubs and flowers and, on one side of the garden, a few vegetables in a bed about 10 by 1.5 metres; it was ideal at the time.

When we moved to Dulverton, the plot was nearly one third of an acre, quite a change. The garden wrapped round the back and both sides of the bungalow, and there were paths all the way around and a large patio, so Lyn was generally able to use either her walker or her scooter, although there were steps up to the patio. Along the perimeters were many established shrubs and trees, which we kept and added to, as they need little maintenance other than a hard prune every year. There was a soft fruit garden, an area used as a potager or small allotment for growing vegetables, and an apple tree and two pear trees. We started growing a few different vegetables for our own use.

Over time, Lyn became unable to get down to weed or plant anything without falling into the beds, which made her laugh—but picking her up was often difficult.

After a couple of years, I built some raised beds, about 600 millimetres high, in the veggie patch, so that Lyn could get close up to weed and help with planting. (The timber for the beds had been free at a large open garden in Devon.) Although the beds were higher, Lyn fell into them occasionally, which she still found amusing…A local builder made the patio more level, removed the original steps and installed a ramp down to the lawn, so Lyn was now able to move around the garden on her scooter.

As Lyn still loved her garden but was less able to tend it, we worked out a system whereby she chose most of the plants, decided which plants should go where, and I did the digging and planting, not a bad compromise. (Lyn always loved a trip to a garden centre, which inevitably included coffee and cake.) She could also use various pots for bulbs and other plants; I would lift them onto a wall or table so that she could work on them while sitting on her rollator or scooter. Another example of finding a way to do something by setting your mind to it.

Lyn also loved sitting in the garden in the sun, looking at the flowers and watching the birds and butterflies on the plants. We created a wildflower and wildlife garden in one area, with a small cast-aluminium table and two chairs in the middle; we called it Tea for Two.

Wisteria was one of Lyn's favourite plants and she was sad to leave one behind when we moved house, so I planted a few in the new garden. Our Harrow Weald wisteria had been growing in a very large tub by the front door for about six years without flowering; we talked to the garden centre staff every year and they always said that it can take several years for a wisteria to establish before flowering. On one occasion, when we complained about it and were told that there was nothing they could do, Lyn said, 'Well, that's not good enough; I want a replacement.'

'Do you have a receipt to prove you bought it from us?' was the reply.

She had already thought of that and produced a six-year-old receipt that she had kept in a drawer. The centre had no choice but to accept it and offered a refund or replacement.

'I want that one,' she said, pointing to a well-established, 2-metre tall tree. That was Lyn.

We had that plant for about three years before we moved and it flowered every year. We went back to the garden centre a few weeks later and there was a prominent sign by the tills that read, 'No plants will be exchanged or replaced over 12 months old.'

I had brought the lawnmower with me to Dulverton but soon after I bought a more powerful petrol mower, as there was such a large area of grass to mow. There would definitely come a time when I would find it difficult so, about seven years ago, we invested in a ride-on mower. I have a great photo of Lyn bestride it—another way she could get involved in the gardening—although she was a little wary of using it.

Lyn loved flower arranging, both at home and creating entries for our local gardening club's flower and produce show; she also arranged a display in one of the local church windows each month. I would go round the garden with her to help cut and collect various types of greenery to go with the flowers she had chosen from our garden or the florist's shop. She also liked doing dried flower arrangements and often gave them as presents to people.

Any form of gardening is good for you, even just a couple of balcony window boxes in a flat. It is uplifting to be out in the fresh air, pottering around and doing what you can. Fresh air and exercise are good for your physical and mental health, and seeing things grow can be very stimulating. Gardening is an excellent activity for anyone, particularly for someone with MS.

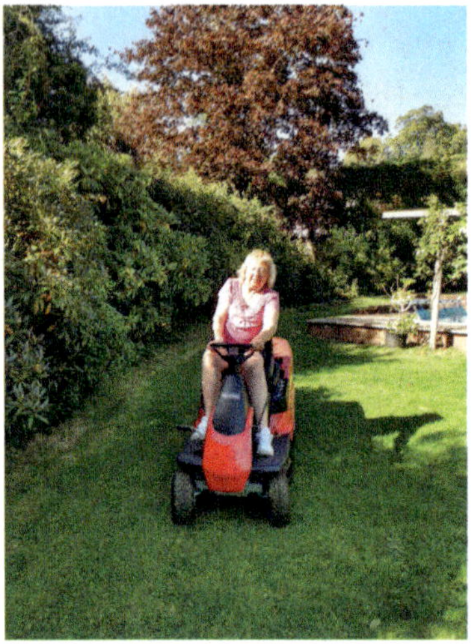

Lyn on ride-on mower.

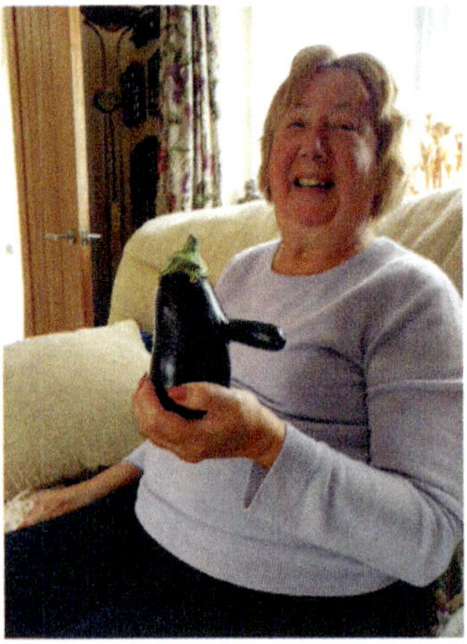

One of our aubergines.

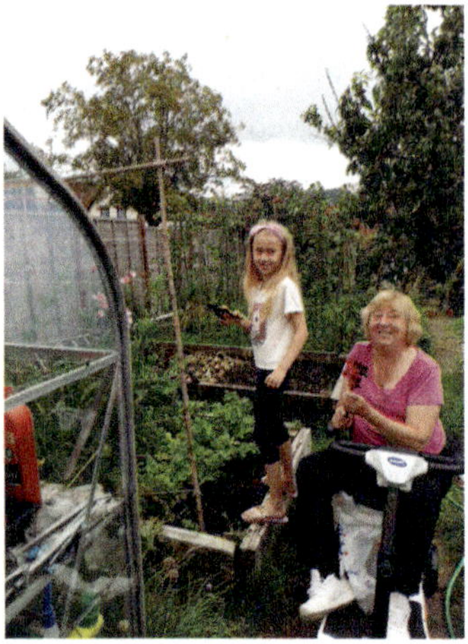

Gardening with Bethany.

36 Scooters

Over the years, Lyn had several rollators, which were very good at the time, and ended up with quite a sturdy, smart one that could fold down. It also had a seat, which was very handy if we were, say, in a friend's garden; she could sit and chat quite happily, then get up and move around, so she used it frequently. The older one stayed at home and she used it when working in the garden she loved, resting when needed.

As Lyn was using a mobility scooter more, we upgraded a few times. First, in Harrow Weald, she had a small lightweight scooter; the steering column could be folded down and the seat removed to allow easier storage in the boot of a car. This was fine, initially, but then something a little sturdier, more reliable, and with a bigger battery for longer distances was required. That also meant an increase in weight, which—with me having to lift it in and out of the boot—was viable for a few years. In fact, we got through four different scooters in ten years.

When we changed Lyn's car five years ago, we also investigated more modern mobility scooters, which might be easier to load into the boot. At the age I was then, I did not know, realistically, how long I could carry on loading and unloading a fairly heavy scooter. We found the ideal version: very sturdy, with a good, modern, long-range battery and, best of all, at the touch of a button, it collapsed to the size of a suitcase. You could then connect it to the straps of a hydraulic lift we had fitted in the boot of the car, push another button and it would rise to a level at which you could simply push it into the boot, drop it level, and lock it in place with its own seatbelt. Brilliant—and it saved my back.

For a while, Lyn was able to stand by the boot, supporting herself on the car body and operate the lift; this was not always easy as trying to balance, support yourself, and operate a remote control all at the same time is not easy for someone with MS.

Lyn always tried to do her best to be as independent as she could and we tried to find things that made this possible. The sad reality is that, as much as the person with MS might want to be independent, this is not always achievable—for any number of reasons. It is a question of doing what, when and how you can, and accepting that, sometimes, you may need help.

If you find you need any kind of mobility aids, have a word with your local MS branch as they may be able to arrange a grant from the MS Society, although Motability should be able to cover most, if not all, of your needs. If you purchase a car though Motability and you need a hoist to lift a scooter in and out of the boot, they can arrange the purchase and install this for you; there may be a small cost for this.

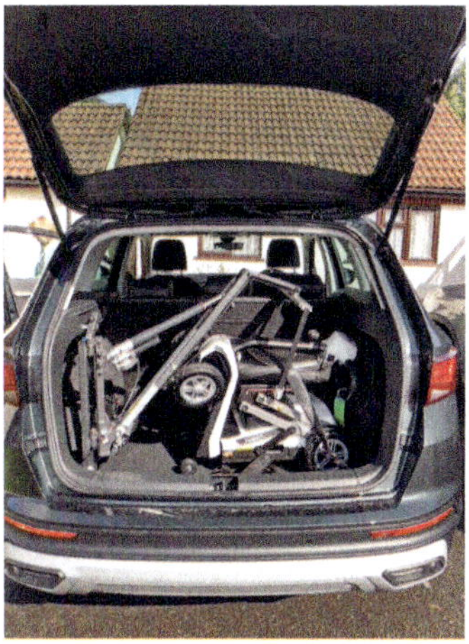

Lyn's new fold-up scooter.

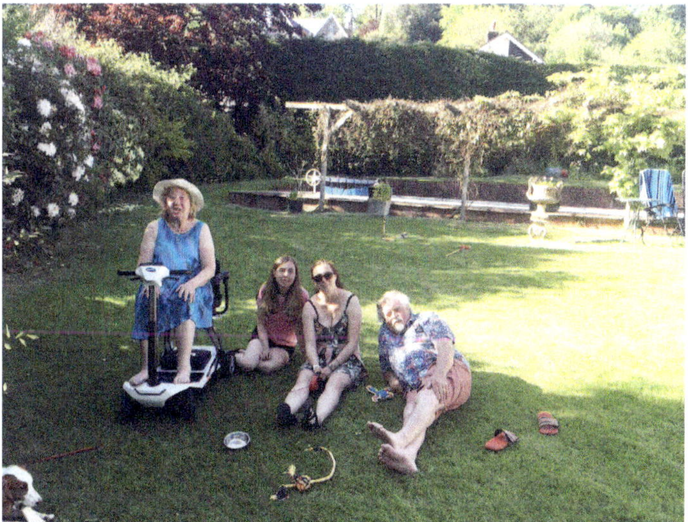

Lyn on her new scooter, chilling in the garden.

37 Symptoms

As time progressed, Lyn's symptoms gradually became worse, as is the case with primary progressive MS. Fatigue was a constant, even after a good night's sleep. Lyn might be fine first thing in the morning but, after a shower, she would feel quite tired and would have to sit down for a while, to recover before getting dressed. The fatigue continued throughout the day; some days were worse than others but it was always there in the background.

We would sometimes go out for a day, with some walking involved; Lyn had started by using my arm or a walking stick to help her balance but later, up to ten years or so after being diagnosed, she started using a walker or rollator. These helped, but she would still tire easily and need to rest. The advantage of a rollator is that they have a seat, so it is easy to rest when you need to; most of them also have a shopping basket under the seat, another very handy feature.

It is a common human trait to want to be active and enjoy yourself; everybody overdoes it now and then but, with MS, you may suffer more than most people afterwards. Lyn would sometimes do something and thoroughly enjoy it, then suffer badly for a few days when her symptoms worsened. But who was I to say, 'No, you can't do that; you know what will happen?' If Lyn wanted to do something, there was not much that stopped her and she just accepted that there might be consequences; all I could do was be there to help pick up the pieces. You cannot stop someone enjoying themselves.

Lyn would still try to walk for short distances as much as she could with her rollator, using her scooter for longer distances; she was not totally reliant on the scooter until 2017/18.

Vertigo

As Lyn's walking became worse, so did her balance; around 2015, tests revealed that she was suffering from vertigo. The NHS website has helpful information on this condition:

> There are loop-shaped canals in your inner ear which contain fluid and fine, hairlike sensors that help you keep your balance. At the base of the canals are the utricle and saccule, each containing a patch of sensory hair cells. Within these cells are tiny particles (otoconia) that help monitor the position of your head in relation to gravity and linear motion, such as going up and down in an elevator or moving forward and backward in a car.

Sometimes crystals develop in these canals and cause an imbalance. There is a procedure called an Epley manoeuvre, a simple, non-invasive approach to treating benign paroxysmal positional vertigo (BPPV), a specific type of vertigo, which a GP can carry out. It involves a series of head movements that help relocate calcium carbonate crystals from your utricle back to your semicircular canals, where they belong. Lyn had this procedure on several occasions and it helped for some time after.

From the NHS website:

There are things you can do to ease vertigo symptoms when

they're happening and to reduce how often it happens.

Do:
Move your head carefully and slowly during daily activities
Lie still in a quiet, dark room to reduce the spinning feeling
Sit down straight away when you feel dizzy
Turn on the lights if you get up at night
Use a walking stick if you are at risk of falling
Sleep with your head slightly raised on 2 or more pillows
Get out of bed slowly and sit on the edge of the bed for a while before standing up
Try to relax–anxiety can make vertigo worse

Don't:
Bend over to pick things up–squat to lower yourself instead
Stretch your neck–for example, while reaching up to a high shelf.

Buzzing

The electrical buzzing sensations in Lyn's hands and sensory issues became gradually worse, but they were always mild, background symptoms. Interestingly, reflexology, a massage that involves applying different amounts of pressure or stimulation to the feet, hands, and ears helped to alleviate these symptoms. It may provide relief for pain, stress and anxiety, among other benefits. Reflexology is based on the theory that your hands, feet, and ears are connected to certain organs and body systems. It is mainly used on the feet, as Lyn's reflexology sessions were.

It is another treatment that has been researched but there is, as yet, little or no scientific basis for its efficacy but it does not cause harm and, if you feel some benefit, why not use it?

Acupuncture works for some people as well. Lyn never tried this as she was a little wary of the needles used. I had a couple of acupuncture courses for my knee, before it was replaced, and I did find that it helped; so, not necessarily for everyone but maybe worth a try?

Speech

Sometimes Lyn's speech would sound slurred which might have made some people think she had had a few too many drinks; this was not the case, of course. She enjoyed a drink or two but too many.

From the MS Society website:

> There are a few different ways MS can cause speech problems.
>
> MS can affect parts of your brain that control the muscles involved in speech. When these muscles are affected, the speech problem is called dysarthria. Some people find that medications they take for MS can contribute to dysarthria.
>
> MS can also affect the messages in the brain that control your voice box. This can change the sound of your voice. It's known as dysphonia.
>
> MS can cause problems with memory and thinking, which can affect communication too. You may have trouble understanding or using language. It can also affect the thought processes involved in communicating. These are sometimes called cognitive communication difficulties.
>
> More rarely, MS can cause specific changes called dysphasia or aphasia.

Clawed toes

One symptom that caused Lyn great deal of a discomfort was clawed toes, which seems to be quite common with MS. It was one of those symptoms that seemed to creep up on her and get worse. It is caused by the tendons under the toes contracting and, if left, can lead to the toes becoming 'frozen'—fixed in one position.

Baclofen, a drug used to treat MS, is a muscle relaxant that works by reducing the transmission of messages between nerve cells. This seems a little odd given that this is what the damage to the myelin sheath causes in the first place. Lyn tried it a couple of times but it made her feel fuzzy headed and slightly nauseous, so she did not take it for long. It seems to work for some people but not others; there are also surgical interventions which you would have to discuss with your health professional.

The clawed toes side effect that caused Lyn discomfort was that her toenails, which had thickened over time—nothing to do with MS—curled under considerably. I tried to cut Lyn's toenails but it was difficult for me with clippers of different kinds, so she needed regular visits to the podiatrist, as he had all the tools to do it properly.

Dexterity

Due to Lyn's dexterity issues, it became difficult, and later almost impossible, for her to do certain things most women take for granted. Finger and toenail care was very difficult for her, so I would do what I could to help. I had always trimmed her fingernails and applied the nail polish but, for some years, she went to a salon. Lyn wanted to look her best and it made her feel good too, which was very important.

Lyn always wanted me to tint her hair, which I was happy to do as there was no way she could do it herself. Her hairdresser jokingly offered me a job as a hair colourist and nail technician.

38 Intimacy in a relationship

If we had asked our two daughters what they thought about their parents' love life, they would probably have said, 'You did it twice, at night, and the lights were off.' Children do not like to think that their parents have a love life. Of course, they may have thought like that in their early teens but have known far better for a long time.

An intimate physical relationship is incredibly important in any marriage or loving relationship; it defines you as a couple. As time progresses, intimacy evolves; we grow older and our intimate relationship changes, for various reasons, even more so when one of you has a disability. The nature and progress of that disability make a significant difference.

I do not know how other couples dealt with this so I can only speak from personal experience. Throughout our lives, we had a very good intimate relationship; there were blips, but that is normal for everyone. MS will always have certain physical and emotional effects on your sexual relationship. The physical effect is obvious as, depending on the level of your disability, certain positions might be difficult, if not impossible. So, you adapt; you find out what feels good—or not—and work out how to change things so that sex can be enjoyable for both of you.

It is not only the physical aspect that changes; the emotional side of any sexual relationship is equally important. But, when you have a physical disability that affects your performance or enjoyment, the emotional side becomes more important. You still need to feel wanted, needed and attractive to your partner, otherwise your sexual relationship becomes meaningless.

There were few things that changed in our sexual relationship, other than some positional changes to make things more enjoyable and comfortable for Lyn, and taking more time with initial arousal—no bad thing for anyone. Lyn needed the reassurance that she was loved and wanted, as she felt she had lost some of her physical attraction. But I was always attracted to her and I still loved her.

There were times when our intimate relationship was far from perfect, which is true for many couples if one of you has a disability, particularly with something like MS, which is not only physical but also affects many aspects of your life. Sometimes, all you need is a kiss and a cuddle.

An intimate relationship is such an important part of life; it is perfectly understandable that, with something like MS, there can be difficulties. Again, communication is key; you must discuss what those difficulties are; if you have a good relationship, you can overcome almost anything.

The MS Society produces an excellent guide on the subject, *Sex and Relationships.*

39 MS and mental health

There are many aspects of MS that can and do impact on your mental health. Lyn sometimes became quite depressed, largely out of a sense of frustration that she could not do what she wanted to do, nor when she wanted. I know, from talking to people with MS and carers, that this is not uncommon. The real problem is that it can be a vicious circle; you feel you cannot do something because you feel tired and that makes you frustrated. You feel anxious, which can lead to stress because you feel you cannot cope with things; the stress makes your symptoms worse, which leads to feeling depressed about the whole thing and the fact that you cannot do anything to change it. That is why it is so important to acknowledge and talk about your feelings. Never bottle things up.

Everyone copes with stress, anxiety and depression in their own way. The MS Society website has excellent information available on these issues:

> The effects of stress
>
> Stress can make you feel anxious or worried, irritable, depressed or low in mood, or a sense of being overwhelmed and becoming very pessimistic. Other common experiences are sleep disturbances and nightmares. Long-term stress can cause physical problems including impaired memory, headaches and high blood pressure.
>
> Stress is a normal part of life for everyone, but in addition to facing normal everyday stresses, people with MS have to

deal with the unpredictability and pressures the condition itself causes. MS can affect many areas of life, such as the ability to work, cognitive functioning, friendships and relationships, housework and parenting.

If all these areas of functioning are being affected by your MS, it is likely you will experience more stress. It is impossible to eliminate stress totally from your life but there are many techniques you can employ to help manage it and take back control.

Ways to manage stress

Learn to recognise what you can and can't control

When you feel stressed, ask yourself 'is this something I have any control over?' If the answer is yes, take any action you know will relieve the stress. It might be something as simple as saying no to your boss. If the answer to your question is no, then 'let go' of the situation that is causing the stress.

Set realistic goals and plan ahead

As MS is unpredictable, having contingency plans in place for everyday activities could reduce stress if the unexpected happens.

Let those who need to know that there is a chance–however small it might be – that the MS could delay your plans.

Is your automatic reaction a true representation of what is happening?

Keep a stress diary for two months. This can help you identify the situations that cause you stress.

Record how you reacted to the difficulty that caused you stress and also how you might have been able to avoid the situation.

Exercise and complementary therapies

This can be a very useful tool in managing stress. Using your body helps to let off steam, releasing stress and anxiety. Exercise also helps with sleep and can give you more energy, both of which can help reduce your stress levels.

Find out more about exercise and MS

Find ordinary everyday activities that are enjoyable to you. Consider complementary therapies like massage, meditation, mindfulness, yoga, t'ai chi or aromatherapy.

Find out more about alternative and complementary therapies

Relaxation and breathing

Teach yourself relaxation and calm breathing techniques. You can buy CDs and books to help you with this, or ask an MS nurse, doctor or other health professional.

Find out more about getting help from a health professional

Anxiety and MS

What is anxiety?

The body's 'fight-or-flight' response is an automatic system that enables us to respond to perceived danger and threats. When we feel fearful or stressed, the body produces adrenaline and this in turn produces physical effects.

These might include a pounding heart, excessive sweating, feeling faint or dizzy, a dry mouth, breathing difficulties, or bowel and urinary problems.

In nature, this physical response can be very useful – it prepares you for immediate action when threatened by danger. But if this heightened state of alertness continues for lengthy periods of time it can affect your health.

Coping with anxiety

The most frequently reported fears from people with MS are around future level of disability.

This is totally understandable, as–even though no one can predict the future, whether they have MS or not–it's very difficult not to worry about it.

Some people get help from professionals to learn how to live with uncertainty, and help them minimise the impact of negative thoughts and feelings on their lives.

Others find strategies like these useful:

Live a day at a time

This doesn't mean putting off planning or burying your head in the sand, but it might mean not thinking the worst will happen tomorrow.

Set a 'worry time'

Make an appointment with yourself to focus on worrying for five minutes each morning and evening. Remember–five minutes–no more and no less.

Write a 'coping with anxiety' list

Put it somewhere you can see it to be reminded of things you can do to help yourself.

Some ideas for what to include:

Identify your fear or anxiety and write it down

Tell someone you trust how you are feeling

Use calming breathing

Do an activity you enjoy to divert yourself

If certain news programmes, magazines, books or people are increasing your fear and anxiety, try to avoid them for a while

Take a relaxing bath

Ask for a hug

Give up smoking (or don't start)

People who smoke often say that it helps them cope with anxiety (and stress). But smoking has been shown to make MS worse. Disability happens at a faster rate, relapsing MS turns into secondary progressive MS sooner, and people who smoke get more lesions and relapses.

In 2021 the biggest ever study into how quitting smoking affects people with MS found two important things.

Anxiety levels were actually higher in people who carried on smoking compared to non-smokers.

Levels of anxiety went down when people quit smoking.

Even better news was that, after quitting, there was a slowing down in how fast their walking and other movement got worse. In fact, the rate it got worse slowed to the same as it is for people who've never smoked.

Signs of depression

If you think you might be depressed, it's important to talk to your health care professional as soon as you can, so you can start to get help. Depression isn't something you can prevent, so you should not feel embarrassed or ashamed of what you are going through.

Your doctor may diagnose you with depression if you have at least five of the following symptoms for at least two weeks:

Depressed mood, feelings of hopelessness and despair
Significantly reduced interest or pleasure in most activities
Changes in appetite and noticeable weight loss or gain
Insomnia (inability to sleep) or hypersomnia (excessive sleeping)
Feelings of excessive restlessness or sluggishness
Fatigue or loss of energy
Feelings of worthlessness, excessive or inappropriate guilt
Reduced ability to think or concentrate, or indecisiveness
Recurrent thoughts of death or suicide

These symptoms would need to be severe enough to upset a daily routine, interfere with relationships, or severely impair work. Health care professionals will also need to establish that the depression is not linked to another cause, such as medication or bereavement.

What causes depression?

There are three main points of view about the causes of depression:

Depression is a medical disease, caused by a neuro-chemical or hormonal imbalance
Depression is caused by certain styles of thinking
Depression is a result of negative experiences

The most commonly held view is that depression is generally caused by some combination of these three factors.

Depression and other MS symptoms

Some symptoms of depression are also symptoms of MS, and it can be difficult to identify what is causing them. For example, fatigue can be related to depression, or may be a direct result of MS, or a combination of the two.

In some conditions there can be a link between being disabled and having depression, but in MS, depression does not seem to be related to how disabled a person is. For example, someone with little physical disability may experience severe depression and vice versa.

There is also no clear link between how long someone has had MS and the risk of being depressed. For example, someone who is recently diagnosed can be as depressed as someone who has had MS for many years.

Nerve damage and depression in MS

Research has been done to see if depression can be directly linked to MS-related damage in particular areas of the brain.

Some studies have suggested that there is a link, though they also suggest that MS-related nerve damage is only part of the equation.

Other factors, including psychological reactions to living with MS, side effects of medication, individual situations and social circumstances are also thought to play a part.

Treatments for depression

If your doctor thinks you might be depressed, they should complete an assessment and draw up a list of factors that may be contributing to it. They should develop a proper depression management strategy, and further assessment, treatment and support should be given.

This might include:

antidepressants - most common are selective serotonin reuptake inhibitors (SSRIs) talking therapies - including psychotherapy and cognitive behaviour therapy (CBT). They can help you develop the 'coping skills' needed to deal with depression-related difficulties. You'll find more about this in our emotional support section.

St John's Wort - might work as well as some antidepressants in mild depression, but not severe. Speak to your GP before taking any complementary medicine.

Lyn was prescribed with Sertraline to help with anxiety and Pregabalin for nerve pain, which is also used to treat anxiety. One of the side effects of both drugs is drowsiness, which she found difficult as she already suffered quite badly with fatigue, so the drowsy feeling did not help. In addition, your body becomes dependent on these drugs, so you cannot simply stop taking them; you have to wean yourself off gradually, following advice from your GP.

If you suffer from any of the above, talk to someone—a family member or friend, initially—to help start the process of dealing with these issues. You may then decide to discuss your concerns with your GP or health professional, with a view to getting a referral to a specialist therapist.

Getting out in the fresh air and doing whatever exercise you can is highly beneficial; in our case, it was walking and swimming. It has been repeatedly proven that exercise, even minimal, is vital for your mental health and overall wellbeing.

40 The Plymouth University VeRMiS Trial

Vestibular Rehabilitation in Multiple Sclerosis, or VeRMiS for short, is the trial that Lyn wanted to be involved with, as it was not age related. This is an extract of the clinical trial parameters from the trial result:

Vertigo, dizziness, poor balance and abnormalities in the control of eye movements are symptoms that may be associated with vestibular problems. Such symptoms are common in people with multiple sclerosis (pwMS), can lead to falls, injury, and a restriction in outdoor mobility, and subsequently may affect social participation and quality of life.

The vestibular system is complex. It consists of the inner ear and vestibular nerve (the peripheral pathways) and pathways in the brain (central pathways) that process information about head and body position. Damage to any of these pathways can result in symptoms of vertigo, dizziness, poor balance and abnormalities of eye movement.

Vestibular rehabilitation (VR) is the standard of care for persons with vestibular problems. VR involves progressive exercises including eye, head, and body movements in sitting, standing, and walking. Given the complexity of symptom presentation in people with MS, such as muscle weakness, spasticity, sensory loss and ataxia, it may be that customised exercises are more effective and cost-effective than home-based generic exercises delivered via a booklet, as is current usual practice.

Although MS affects the central nervous system, approximately 50% of cases of vertigo are caused by a condition called benign paroxysmal positional vertigo (BPPV). In these cases, calcium carbonate crystals from part of the inner ear (otoliths) become dislodged and enter into another part of the inner ear (semi-circular canal) causing symptoms of vertigo on certain head and body movements. BPPV can be diagnosed and treated at the bedside using specific manoeuvres that aim to move these crystals back into position. Currently these testing and repositioning manoeuvres for BPPV are not routinely performed in pwMS and the success and re-occurrence rates are unclear.

The VeRMiS study will involve 140 ambulant pwMS who present with vertigo and/ or dizziness across two study centres: Plymouth and London, UK. Participants who are able to take part will attend an initial assessment and then be enrolled in to one of two trial based upon the assessment findings.

Trial one: A pragmatic multi-centre randomised controlled trial to compare the clinical and cost effectiveness of a 12 week customised VR programme vs generic VR.

Trial two: An observational study to determine the success and re-occurrence rate of BPPV symptoms with repositioning manoeuvres.

A range of outcomes, including self-report and clinical tests of dizziness, mobility and quality of life will be measured at intervals throughout the study.

That is the clinical explanation; this is what happened. The trial involved an in initial assessment at the University in Plymouth for about half a day, during which Lyn had to undergo many tests to assess her ability to deal with various things that affected her walking, balance, movement and cognitive issues. It was a blind trial lasting twelve weeks; one group would see a physiotherapist weekly, while the other group followed the same exercises online, and the results would be compared. Lyn took part in the trial by seeing a physiotherapist once a week at the MS therapy centre in Exeter.

It started in October 2019, just before the pandemic, fortunately, otherwise it would not have happened. It was due to finish in January 2020. At this time Lyn could still use her walking stick and a rollator, supplemented by a scooter for longer distances. The exercises would have been impossible, had she not been as mobile as she was at that time. Although Lyn did all the exercises herself, the physiotherapist and I were always in the background, in case she overbalanced. It was challenging for her, as she had to confront certain fears that had increased as her MS had developed. She had to go through a series of specific exercises on the day, one each week, and she continued the exercises at home the following week.

I would help Lyn repeat the exercises so, by the time of the next session, she could confidently demonstrate that the exercises had worked and she could progress to the next stage. It was a case of repeating the exercises and noting how certain things improved over time.

Lyn was quite focused during this period and she kept up the different exercises, which could be quite challenging. For example, people with MS tend to be very wary when walking and constantly look down, as they need to know that they are walking on the level and where the trip hazards might be. You and I would walk along a pavement and see what was ahead; when you are near a kerb, you know it is there and you step over it. Someone with MS has to constantly look down at the kerb as they approach it and walk over it, ever mindful of the fact that one foot had to stay on the kerb while the other one dropped over it. They have to try to maintain balance with one foot in mid air, while holding a walking stick—without over-balancing. It is very difficult to explain that scenario to anyone who has not experienced being fearful of losing balance and falling over.

The exercises included:

Without a walking stick, standing on the spot, focusing on something in the distance and trying to maintain your balance.

Trying the same sequence again but with your eyes closed.

Trying the same sequence again and then touching your nose with your fingertip.

Walking in a straight line, looking straight ahead, then doing it again while stepping onto a step, walking a few paces, then turning around and doing the same thing again.

Standing on a foam-filled bag with your legs apart to start with, and maintaining your balance while focusing ahead, then gradually bringing your feet closer together to challenge your balance.

Lying down on your back on a raised bed, then sitting up moving to one side, dropping your feet to the floor and standing up straight; not easy if your balance is off.

Standing and holding your balance while watching a video of people going up and down escalators, or a video simulating you moving along the aisles in a supermarket with people coming towards you, or, simulating you walking through a tube station concourse, going up the stairs to the top while people are constantly moving around you.

All these exercises were deliberately designed to challenge fears about balance and vertigo increasingly through the trial. After Lyn went through these exercises at home, between the weekly sessions with the physiotherapist, we had to keep a daily record of the amount of time she could do a particular exercise and how frequently.

With practice at home, her balance and posture did noticeably improve during the trial and she continued with some of them daily, even when the trial finished, as they helped her. Based on our experience, I would say that if the exercises from this trial were available generally for people with MS, they would be beneficial; they certainly were for Lyn. It will be interesting to see which benefits are indicated when the trial results are published. This is what is known to date:

Vestibular rehabilitation can benefit people with **multiple sclerosis (MS)** by addressing symptoms related to balance, dizziness, and vertigo. Here's how it works:

Improved Balance: Vestibular exercises help enhance balance control, reducing the risk of falls.

Reduced Dizziness: Customized exercises target the

vestibular system, minimizing dizziness and vertigo.

Enhanced Eye-Head Coordination: VR improves eye-head coordination, crucial for daily activities.

Adaptation and Compensation: The brain learns to adapt to vestibular deficits and compensate for them.

From my own observations of how Lyn coped with the exercises, I think a person with MS would be more likely to benefit from the weekly sessions with the physiotherapist than from following online instructions. Someone with MS has confidence in the physiotherapist's ability to help guide them through the exercises by ensuring that they are in the right positions. The physiotherapist is not allowed to physically support you or put you in a specific position; you have to attempt it yourself to benefit.

41 Covid-19 and lockdown

Like everyone, we were affected by the Covid-19 pandemic. We were fortunate to have booked a two-week holiday in Barbados for the middle of February 2020; we had a very good holiday and, as always, the warm weather did Lyn good. She was always able to function so much better in warm weather, particularly walking; she could still manage short distances either holding my arm or using her walking stick, although she still had to use her rollator for walks of any distance. We had to hire a car to travel around, as Barbados is not renowned for its accessible pavements or transport so she could not have used her scooter.

Within weeks of arriving home, there were news items about a virus spreading in China; on 23 March, the UK Government announced the introduction of a national lockdown. In common with most of the population, we could not go anywhere at first, other than limited essential journeys; during those initial months, we lived out of the freezer. Fortunately, we had a large chest freezer in the utility room and a small one in the kitchen under the fridge. For years, I had made double portions of dishes such as curries, casseroles and sauces, which, together with frozen meat, chicken and fish, and frozen garden vegetables, meant that we could have been almost self-sufficient for six months or more. All we needed was fresh fruit and vegetables and toiletries. Even when the shops began reopening under strict conditions, I would not let Lyn go anywhere them for at least the first three months, as I did not want to risk exposing her unnecessarily to infection.

Covid-19 is still here and always will be, in its many potential variants, but as of August 2024, seventy per cent of the world population has had at least one dose of the vaccine and travel has opened up. If you have MS, you have the same risk of developing Covid-19 as anyone. People with MS are at no greater risk than the general public of becoming infected with this particular coronavirus; MS does not weaken your immune system. An exception to this is if you are taking certain disease-modifying drugs, some of which suppress parts of your immune system, leaving you at a greater risk of infection. If you are concerned, do check with your MS nurse or neurologist. You should not stop any treatment or miss appointments until you've spoken to a health professional.

For that entire first year, we hardly went anywhere; once it was permitted, we started to drive a little further and take Lyn's scooter and I would walk where there were very few or no people. We did not go to the hairdresser; it was a good year before we went and, at first, we had to wear a mask. Our hairdresser, Emma, had to wear a full-face shield and could have only one client in the salon at a time.

Lyn's hair grew considerably but my hair always grew faster and thicker; after a year it was like being back in the 1970s—it was past my shoulders. I became used to it so have kept it longish ever since.

One of the worst things I remember was, driving to our daughter, Sarah, in Winterbourne, Bristol, just before Christmas 2020, about a two-hour journey. We had to park in the driveway to drop off presents and then just wave and blow kisses to her, Steve and our grandchildren,

Matt and Will. There were many tears on the way home that day.

If that were not bad enough, our other daughter, Kelly, her husband, Keith, and grandchildren, Hayden and Bethany, live in Leighton Buzzard, which is four hours' drive away. We did not see them until 2021, which was very upsetting.

This whole period was so hard for Lyn, as her family was always the most important thing to her and not being able to visit them or have them visit us was incredibly hard for us both. Thank God for WhatsApp videos on mobile phones and laptops and Zoom on laptops and PCs; they made life a little easier as we could at least communicate and see each other. I shudder to think what it would have been like if the pandemic had hit in, say, the 1980s, 1990s or even the early 2000s; the technology did not exist to enable that kind of communication. The effects on the population, government and businesses would have been catastrophic.

What did we do in lockdown? That is a question everyone still asks. The pandemic affected so many working people in so many ways, unless you were a key worker you could not travel to work or meet people. I could not do any architectural work as I could not travel to see clients; council planning offices and building control departments closed down and, when they resumed working, their staff were working from home. I did little work for at least twelve to eighteen months. Being self-employed, I could not furlough myself and I could not claim benefits so, like many people I had to live off my savings.

We spent some of the time catching up on things we

had put on the back burner for a few years, such as sorting out photos. I caught up with some artwork, painting in watercolour and acrylic, and practising my guitar playing. Lyn had taken up enamelling; a friend had introduced her to it a few years earlier. It meant applying the powdered glass to copper or other suitable metal, then fusing them together at high temperature in a kiln oven. I always stayed close at hand when Lyn was either putting something in the oven or taking it out; I could not contemplate leaving her to do it on her own and sometimes she wanted me to do it for her. She started making jewellery like earrings and brooches and I have since decided to try it myself, using Lyn's materials and equipment.

Like so many others, we also binge-watched programmes on Netflix, Prime Video and iPlayer. Under normal circumstances, I probably would not have watched most of the period dramas but Lyn enjoyed them and so did I, to a degree.

As the effects of the pandemic eased, we returned very slowly and warily to travelling for shopping; it was a break from the normality we all seemed to have settled into and we looked forward to it. As soon as it was allowed, we started to travel but, initially, only to see our families, which was so good after being unable to for so long. Even though travel restrictions were lifted, we never went abroad again as we did not want to risk getting Covid-19. One of the main reasons was that, as Lyn's MS had worsened and I was still her only carer, I did not want to be laid up with the virus, unable to look after her.

42 Catheter and sepsis

Lyn's bladder control had been bad for several years, to the extent that she used incontinence pants every day and night. This involved changes around the clock, sometimes at home, sometimes when we were out, which all took some dealing with. Helping her change was a regular occurrence; it was part of our everyday life.

We talked to the GP, the consultant and the specialist nurse and after several years of discussion, discomfort, embarrassment and NHS waiting lists, Lyn decided to have a Supra Pubic Catheter fitted, which would enable her to control her bladder by using a day bag and night bag. After having the catheter fitted, it is normal to use a bag to drain it, as you only have to empty the day bag in the evening and swap it for the night bag. It is possible to use a valve tap and tube and empty your bladder directly into the toilet, which is fine for a man but not so good for a woman, for whom a bag is the easiest option. You also have to keep an eye out for leaks, as the tube can bend or come undone.

In mid-November 2021, Lyn was admitted to Musgrove Park Hospital in Taunton for the operation. A few days later, after returning home, she was so ill that I called the GP, who attended very quickly, suspected that she had a nasty infection, and they called for an ambulance. She was admitted to hospital and diagnosed with full-blown sepsis and blood tests revealed that she now also had type 2 diabetes. Sepsis would knock the stuffing out of anyone, let alone someone with MS; it made her symptoms much worse and she never really recovered.

Lyn returned home after a few days, but she was never the same and I could sense that things were getting worse. As well as her normal daily care, I now had to monitor her blood sugar levels and give her daily insulin injections.

In December 2021, I suffered the worst pain I had ever experienced—unable to pee or poo. I had an initial triage call from the GP, then an appointment. He examined me and suggested an enema, which I tried but, on day three, the pain was so intense that I called again and he booked me into Musgrove Park's acute medical unit. This was problematic as I could not leave Lyn on her own, and I did not know if I would be admitted. I called our daughter, Sarah, who was nearest, but she could not come to stay with Lyn as she had contracted Covid-19. Thankfully, Chris, a good friend of ours, said she could stay with Lyn until our daughter, Kelly, and husband, Keith, travelled down from Leighton Buzzard. They would stay with Lyn overnight and for as long as possible, as Keith's mother could look after Hayden and Bethany.

When the A&E staff examined me, they found that my bladder was in retention; they inserted a catheter and drained off a couple of litres of fluid. What a relief that was! I had suffered kidney failure, as everything had backed up with nowhere to go; a scan showed that I had a benign enlarged prostate, so I would have to have a catheter inserted and use a leg bag for the foreseeable future until the prostate could be treated. Luckily, I was only in hospital for three days and came back to take over from Kelly.

When I reached home Kelly's first words to me on the doorstep were, 'How the fuck have you managed to keep looking after Mum the last few months without help? I've only looked after her for a few days and I'm exhausted.'

When you are the carer, you just carry on dealing with things as you always have; as things worsen, you adapt and do not think about it. It is only when someone outside of the normal routine steps in to help that you realise how bad things are. They notice the step changes that you had not. Kelly did not realise how much and how quickly Lyn's symptoms had worsened as none of us had seen as much of each other as we used to pre-pandemic. Frankly, neither had I—I was just dealing with things as normal. I must admit that, for some weeks before I went into hospital, as Lyn's symptoms worsened considerably, I had been struggling—getting her ready in the mornings, helping her to shower, dress and get ready for the day, helping her with her needs during the day, and then helping her get ready for bed at night. I realised that I now needed help… to help Lyn.

I had enquired locally and a few trusted friends recommended a lady called Hannah. Although Covid-19 had prevented Sarah from coming down, she managed to contact Hannah, who was available to help in the mornings. Sarah arranged for her to have an initial meeting with us. A few days after I came home, we met Hannah and Lyn immediately felt very comfortable with her, which was very important to both of us; Hannah started the next morning. Over the next few days, we settled into a routine; Lyn felt at ease with Hannah and the help she gave Lyn with showering and dressing took some of the load off me.

I still had to help Lyn during the day and then get her ready for bed at night.

During this time I noticed that Lyn's overall condition was worsening. The cause of the onset of secondary progressive MS is still unclear, even to expert medical professionals, as it can vary from one person to another, in terms of cause, effect or time. Medical evidence does point towards secondary progressive MS developing from relapsing remitting, but not from primary progressive, and doctors require more evidence over a period of time as to whether or not secondary progressive has developed or is developing. There is also plenty of anecdotal evidence that something causes an 'infection', which can cause a significant deterioration in the symptoms, from which a person never seems to fully recover and which can progress into secondary progressive MS. Generally speaking, medical specialists are unable to diagnose secondary MS with any certainty until six months or so after an 'attack' as a certain amount of time and observation has to elapse. I can remember instances of friends with MS, either relapsing remitting or primary progressive, who have had an attack of some kind, or another illness, and have suddenly gone downhill, never to fully recover.

Could the sudden decline have been associated with Lyn's sepsis episode or was it something else? With all this in mind, I felt that I was staring down the barrel at secondary progressive developing. Lyn's physicality had changed since the bout of sepsis and her balance was affected. She found it increasingly difficult to walk without me helping her or using her walker indoors; sometimes she would even sit in it so that I could push her around the bungalow. Her fatigue was increasing and she used to nap frequently during the day. It could be that it was not secondary progressive developing but the early symptoms of something else.

43 The hospital

On Saturday, 18 December 2021, we decided to get a wheelchair for Lyn to use indoors, so that I could help her move around more easily, and she used it that weekend. On the morning of 20 December, after Hannah had finished getting her ready, I noticed a slight yellowing on the skin of Lyn's forehead. This worried me so I called the GP; he saw Lyn at home and said he was concerned that she had developed jaundice, so he called for an ambulance to take her to Musgrove Park A&E. It arrived early evening and the crew said I should stay home and call the hospital in the morning. When I called, I learned that Lyn had been admitted to a ward so I went to the hospital to spend time with her. She had some tests and a scan that day but, by 6.00pm, the scan results were still not available so I went home and asked the hospital to call me later.

At about 8.00pm, I received a call, asking me to come in at 9.00pm to meet one of the doctors. I went back in trepidation and waited in Lyn's room for the registrar. When she arrived, she told us that the scan had shown that Lyn had an inoperable tumour on her pancreas; there was no cure—it would end her life. Lyn would have months rather than years and palliative care was the only option. The registrar explained what to expect and the care and help that would be available; they would carry out a procedure to insert a stent to lift the tumour off the pancreas. This would enable bile to flow again, which would alleviate the jaundice symptoms.

I looked down at Lyn, who had had a pretty rough couple of days; she was barely awake, let alone in any condition to take in the enormity of what the doctor was telling us. 'You are not getting any of this,' was my only thought.

After the doctor left, it was obvious Lyn was in a deep sleep so I decided to come back in the morning. During the drive home, I made my two hardest telephone calls ever to Sarah and Kelly, to tell them that their mum had a terminal illness. They were understandably devastated and we all shed many tears that evening. I did not get much sleep that night and dreaded the next day.

At the hospital the next morning, I found Lyn sitting in bed wide awake and smiling; we had some coffee and I asked her if the doctors had been round. She said that they had mentioned doing a procedure but she was not sure what it was. I then had to do the most difficult thing I had ever done; I had to tell the love of my life everything the doctor had told me.

'Am I going to die?'

'Yes, my darling; we just don't know when.'

'But I've got so much I want to do.'

We shed so many tears that day, interspersed with talking to the doctors and nurses, as we tried to comprehend what was happening and how things would progress.

It was the worst day of my life, having to have that conversation with Lyn, then dealing with the practicalities of the diagnosis and planning what would happen Deeply upset as I was, I knew that, while I was with Lyn each day, I had to stay strong for her; my tears could wait until I got home.

At that time, the hospital had a fairly open visiting time and Sarah and Kelly were able to stay with me and we visited Lyn in a shift system. Weeks before Christmas, we had already planned that Sarah and Kelly would spend Christmas Day at their homes, with their children, and travel down on Boxing Day to stay with us for a few days.

When we knew what was happening to Lyn, we discussed it and decided to carry on with the original plan, so that it would not upset the grandchildren. Sarah and Kelly would still be able to visit Lyn, in turn with me.

Sarah drove down to the hospital at about 10.00am on Christmas Day and I met her in reception an hour later, having called her when I arrived, as Lyn was allowed only one visitor in her room at a time. Sarah came out smiling and said that Lyn's consultant had said she could go home to be with her family on Boxing Day. At that point, the doctor arrived in reception and I could have kissed him—but made do with a handshake. He said he would make the arrangements; all we had to do was collect Lyn.

I discussed it with Sarah and Kelly and we agreed that Steve, Keith and I would leave as soon as possible on Boxing Day morning to collect Lyn, as it would need the three of us to safely transfer her from the wheelchair to the car and back again later. We drove up together, all wearing Santa Claus hats; we kidnapped Lyn and took her home for what would be her last Christmas with us. She stayed from 11.30am to 4.30pm, by which time she was very tired, but at least she had been home for a Christmas with her grandchildren, which she loved. There were plenty of smiles and much laughter while she was home and we managed to take some very special photos.

Lyn could manage only a small amount of food for lunch, but she still had room for some Christmas pudding and cake, which was par for the course. It was a wonderful few hours of normality in a far from normal situation. Steve and Keith helped me take Lyn back and I got her settled in for the night.

Over the next few days the girls were able to visit Lyn but, on New Year's Eve, the hospital decided to go into lockdown as there had been several Covid cases among the staff and patients. No visitors were allowed.

As I was Lyn's full-time carer as well as her husband, the ward sister agreed that I could come for as long as I wanted during the day to help look after her, as long as I stayed in the hospital while I was there. At least I was free to go to the on-site M&S for a sandwich or something Lyn fancied as a treat. For the next five weeks I would arrive at the hospital at 10.00am and stay until about 6.30pm, sitting with Lyn, chatting, helping with her personal care, showering or washing, getting her ready in the morning, helping her go to the toilet, changing, helping her eat and drink, and getting her ready for bed—all that I had been doing at home. I am not sure what the nurses made of this, initially, but, after a few days, we soon fell into a routine whereby I could look after the non-medical care and be there for Lyn, while they got on with their medical tasks. It worked well.

I cannot imagine how I could have dealt with this situation if it had happened during the pandemic, when I would not have been allowed into the hospital to help with Lyn's care. Like many other hospital patients at the time, she might have given up. At least I can be thankful that I had the opportunity to look after her while she was in hospital, something which hundreds of people, possibly thousands, were not permitted to do. I could not fault the doctors, nurses and health care assistants who helped Lyn; they all did what they could to make her comfortable and always treated her with dignity and respect.

During the first two weeks the doctors tried to get Lyn's jaundice under control, which was difficult as the tumour on her pancreas prevented the bile flowing and was causing the jaundice. On the second attempt, a stent was successfully inserted and, within a week, her jaundice symptoms were alleviated, which made her more comfortable.

I am forever grateful that we took the decision, all those years earlier, to travel as much as we could afford to, visit as many countries as possible, and do what we could. There was never any certainty about how Lyn's MS would affect her in the future and limit what she could do. Now we were faced with something that was nothing to do with MS and which would end her life, so it made that decision even more important.

Lyn's appetite had decreased since she had come into hospital; she was not eating much at all, although she did manage small amounts, predictably some of the desserts, such as rice pudding or custard.

We had many photos and videos from our travels and I was able to take those to the hospital on the laptop—to relive those memories on a series of compilations.

There was much laughter, as well as tears, in those weeks; we looked at the photos and videos and watched old comedy films that she loved, including the Marx

Brothers, Ealing comedies, *Fawlty Towers*, and *Notting Hill*.

We were talking one afternoon, about things we would like to do.

'What would you still like to do, now, if you had the chance?' I asked.

Lyn thought for a minute.

'I'd like to be back in Barbados in the sun sitting on a beach with you, with a glass of bubbly in one hand and a big spliff in the other,' she replied. That was my girl.

Because Lyn always felt better for having her nails done, I took in some of her favourite nail polishes, trimmed and sanded her nails, and put on what would be the last nail polish she would have applied. She always wanted to look her best.

Towards the end of January, it became obvious that Lyn's condition was worsening. We had a discussion with her consultant, who said that there was another procedure they could possibly do, but it would mean transferring to a hospital in Bristol for a couple of days. There was obviously no guarantee of any improvement; it would just extend her life for a time. We had discussed long before this current diagnosis that, if either of us were in this position and there was no clear benefit to having an invasive procedure, in these circumstances it should not be carried out. This decision was made easier by the fact that, since being diagnosed with pancreatic cancer five weeks earlier she had never actually been in any pain, something I was very thankful for; she just wanted quality of life for how ever long was left. We talked this over with the consultant and, in the end, Lyn said, 'I just want to go home.'

There were a few hurdles to overcome and the hospital

administration staff were not as helpful as they could have been. The last few days were made worse by bureaucracy, which I will not go into here as it would detract from the excellent medical care that Lyn had received. The greatest challenge was getting care in place at home for Lyn; I asked the administration staff simply to organise whatever needed doing to get her home and that I would pay for it. This shifted the ground somewhat, as they would not have to pay for the care or the carers, although I would have to organise them.

They arranged for a hospital bed, all the equipment we would need, and all the essential medication to be in place when we arrived home. I did have difficulty trying to organise the care package and, in desperation on the Thursday morning, I called Hannah. I told her what I needed and it was as if she had been waiting for my call... She could start helping with end of life care for Lyn the day after we were home—29 January 2022.

44 At home for the last week

There is no doubt that this was a very tough time for our whole family, particularly Sarah, Kelly and me. Sarah arranged to stay with me for as long as needed, while Steve stayed at home with their children, Matt and Will, who were fourteen and eleven at the time. Kelly was able to come down with Keith, as his parents could look after Hayden and Bethany.

We had a discussion with Hannah about Lyn's end of life care; because she had cared for her previously, they had talked about all sorts of things and she had a good understanding of Lyn as a person and of her feelings. She recommended an holistic approach, which not only provides high quality care, it also makes the end of life process easier for both patients and their loved ones by meeting the patient's spiritual, social and emotional needs.

We got into a routine whereby Sarah and Kelly took on the support role to Hannah, doing what I had done for Lyn at home and in the hospital, while I would be in the background and helping with turning and lifting and comforting Lyn, while the girls helped with her personal care. They were more than willing to do this for their mum, though it was difficult for them seeing her like that. Sarah and Kelly helped care for Lyn with all the love, kindness and attention that only daughters can give. At least Lyn was now home in her happy place surrounded by the love of her family.

We wanted Lyn's last days to be in as normal a family

environment as possible, so we set up her bed in the living room where she could be in the middle of everything, look out at the garden, and see the plants and birds that she had always loved. We had the TV on for whatever Lyn wanted to watch or Alexa for background music, playing all the songs she loved.

Understandably, Lyn did not feel like eating much, just porridge for breakfast, a little soup for lunch, and maybe some rice pudding or custard later. Although I was still treating her diabetes, she liked mostly sweet things: Lucozade, banana milkshakes, Coca-Cola and ice pops; not exactly a diabetic diet but she enjoyed it.

Lyn's brother, Peter, and her niece, Amy, visited, as did some of our friends; there was plenty of humour and laughter at times, particularly on the Saturday before she passed away, when she seemed to join in with everything going on around her.

On the Sunday, Lyn fell into a deep sleep, from which she never truly woke. Sarah, Kelly and I took turns to sit with her that night, as we sensed it would not be long. Lyn's breathing changed around 5.30am on Monday and we were all there holding her, stroking and kissing her face and telling her how much we loved her. It was all very peaceful and, thankfully, she had never been in any pain.

Lyn suddenly opened her eyes and turned towards me; as she took her last breath, my face was the last thing she saw. Lyn passed away at 6.05am on Monday 7 February, 2022.

45 Lyn's funeral

We planned Lyn's funeral for 24 February at our local church, All Saints' in Dulverton. We invited as many of our family and friends that could make it and they filled the church.

The service was perfect, exactly what Lyn would have wanted, her favourite hymns and psalms and two pieces of music that she loved, *Canto de la Terra*, by Andrea Bocelli, as processional music, and Lionel Richie's *Three Times a Lady* as the recessional music. When we were planning the service our rector, the Reverend Dowell Conning, had asked about our choice of music. He said that there would not be a dry eye in the house—and he was right.

Lyn had always loved colour in its many forms, so we asked everyone to wear something colourful, which was a joy to see on such a sad occasion.

After the service, we held a wake at the town hall, which was attended by many family and friends. We had spent a great deal of time choosing photos of Lyn, from her childhood to the end of her life; our friend, Gerry, put these onto the digital projector and they were displayed, on a loop, on a large screen on the stage. It was so good to have so many people there and it was a chance for family and friends to meet each other, talk about Lyn and what she meant to them, and enjoy and laugh at the photos.

It was a very sad day but there were many lighter moments at the wake, as well; Lyn had a good send-off, which she would have loved.

46 Grief

'Grief is the price we pay for love.'
Colin Murray Parkes

Grief is very personal and everyone reacts to it in their own way. You feel anger and frustration; it is frightening, you sometimes feel as if you have no control over your emotions and it can be all consuming. The anger you feel is against the world and everyone in it. Why did not the doctors and the hospital do more? Did I do enough over the years; could I have done more?

The person you love most has passed away. Why? What did she do to deserve that? If there is a God, why did he take her? It was all too soon…

It takes a long time to process all this. Anger means hitting out at anything and everything that you can possibly blame for what has happened; it is illogical but you are not thinking logically, you are lashing out because you are angry at what has happened, and frustrated that there is nothing you can do about it. The reality is that the doctors and the nurses did all that they could, and could not have done any more; they cared for her and carried out whatever treatments Lyn needed. The palliative care nurses talked with us and tried to provide us with whatever information we might need to deal with what was happening. But, while you are grieving, none of this matters; you are somehow blind to it.

Yes, I did do enough; I could not have done more than

I did and that was enough, but, after more than two years since Lyn passed away, sometimes I still feel all of these things. Someone once said to me that it can take two to five years to reach the point where the person you have lost is not the first thing you think of in the morning when you wake. That is about right.

At night, in the silence before I go to bed, I have sat on the sofa, thought about Lyn and cried ceaselessly. I have said how much I miss her, how much I still love her. I have stood looking out at the garden and shouted and screamed and asked why. In that first year, there were few days when I did not cry, and there have been many similar days since. Something sets me off—a song on the radio, something someone says; there are so many triggers. But there have also been many occasions when I have smiled or laughed at something that I know Lyn would have felt the same about; it is not all sadness.

Sarah and Kelly say that they have felt the same.

I still say good morning or goodnight to Lyn or talk to her during the day when I think of something she would have liked. I have always been open with my emotions; I cry with pride at some of the things my grandchildren do that Lyn will never see, but I sense that she is there, watching over us all. I cry seeing new-born babies, hearing about illnesses that affect young children and their fight for life, stories of people taking on amazing fundraising challenges, even though they are suffering themselves. I believe it is the deep love I still have in my heart for Lyn that brings all these thoughts to the surface.

What you begin to realise, as time goes by, is that it is absolutely fine to feel all these things; it is completely normal. Grief is something you never truly get over, you just learn to live with it and deal with it day by day.

I have always found it very easy to talk to people and I know I can talk to my family and friends; they will listen and simply let me talk about how I feel and my memories of Lyn. Some people find it difficult to express their feelings and emotions, but it is far better for your own mental health to talk about them, if not to family and friends, maybe to a counsellor; talking is good.

One thing you never fully understand, until it happens to you, is the year of firsts after your life partner has passed: the first birthday, the first anniversary, the first Christmas—without them. These special dates can be particularly difficult; fortunately, I had the comfort of Sarah and Kelly either being with me or, at a distance, on FaceTime.

I still celebrate each significant date, just as we would have done together. I go somewhere that we used to visit for the day, have lunch where we used to, and raise a glass in her memory.

Lyn had a very simple faith; she believed in God and would go to church when she could. We were both christened and confirmed and I would go with her. We also had beliefs from other religious traditions, which made sense to us, not have one single faith but a blend of faiths. When we lived in Harrow Weald, Lyn told a vicar that she would like to come back as a bird.

'You are in the wrong religion,' was his response.

I don't know if Lyn has come back as a bird but I do know that, on many occasions, I have been woken by the same bird flying to the window, tapping at it, and staying there until I have gone to see it. Or, I might be walking or sitting somewhere; a bird will alight on a bush and stay there, even when I am quite close. It always seems to be a robin. Sarah and Kelly have had similar experiences.

Every now and then a little white feather will appear out of nowhere…One day, not long after Lyn passed, I was walking in the garden and, as I turned, there was a white dove on the path. It walked to within a couple of feet of me, then slowly took off. A sign her spirit was there? I do not know, but I did feel something I am unable to explain.

I do not know if that was a message of some kind but some religions believe that birds are messengers of spirits. There is still so much that I do not understand and probably never will, but I think that your beliefs give you comfort and that can only be to the good.

The main thing I have been doing to deal with and channel my grief positively is to write this book; it has been very cathartic to clear my mind and not dwell on the sadness, but to celebrate Lyn's life and her love of life. I hope it will help others.

It was the Reverend Dowell Conning who was instrumental in this; a few days after conducting Lyn's funeral, he suggested that, as part of the grieving process, I might find it helpful to keep a diary of my thoughts and feelings. I did that for a few months and, shortly afterwards, I had the idea of writing a book.

Memory is a strange thing. In writing this, I have found that I have moved from one chapter to another, as something I write always brings another memory to the surface, be it sad or funny. Few people get the chance to do this so I am grateful for the opportunity of setting things down for others to read, hopefully enjoy, and maybe gain something from it. I would love my grandchildren to read this one day, to help them remember their Nana as the wonderful person she was.

47 Life after Lyn

In the first few weeks after Lyn passed away, I spent much time dealing with all the necessary paperwork and planning her funeral with Sarah and Kelly. For anyone going through this process, the paperwork is now far easier than ever; it is, essentially, a one-stop shop. Once a death is registered, you arrange for a form to be issued by the registrar, who then notifies all the necessary government departments and they then contact you. It certainly removes much of the stress.

This way of dealing with the paperwork was one of the few positive things to emerge from the pandemic; it was introduced out of necessity—to limit personal contact.

Lyn had always said she wanted a service at our local church, which she had attended over the years, and she wanted to be cremated. She could never make up her mind what should happen to her ashes so I made an executive decision, one of the few that she was not involved in, that half of her ashes would be interred in our local churchyard and half would be scattered at the crematorium where her mother's ashes were scattered. I had managed to find out the grid reference of the exact location.

Some weeks after Lyn's funeral, I started to return to some kind of normality. For about six years before Lyn passed away, as her MS symptoms worsened, I stopped taking on work on that was not local, say within one hour's drive and only for two to three days a week. This was mainly to enable us to spend more time doing what we wanted to do together, whether simply spending time with each other, travelling abroad or going on day trips in the car, which she loved. After she passed away, I have continued with that work; I still had to occupy my time, do something to keep my brain going, meet people, and I enjoyed it. I still paint, play the guitar, and meet family and friends; in other words, more or less what I used to do. There was more reason to do so than not. Your brain is a complex organ but, just like a muscle, if you do not use it, you lose it, and I do not want that to happen. If Lyn had thought I was sitting around moping she would have kicked my backside.

Lyn was the only woman I knew who had three engagement rings. After her fingers swelled up some years ago, the original ring I bought her no longer fitted and, due to its design, could not be resized. The first time we went to Barbados, we were looking in a Holetown jewellery shop, where Lyn saw an emerald ring.

'Oh, that's lovely,' she said, and tried it on. It was like Cinderella's slipper; it fitted perfectly.

'So, would you like that?' I asked. Silly question, really; of course she did, so I bought it.

Some years later, when we were in Sri Lanka, Lyn spotted a fine sapphire ring in a jewellery shop.

'Oh, that's lovely,' she said. It was Cinderella's slipper all over again, another perfect fit, so I bought that as well. For ever after, she would wear whichever ring worked with her outfit for the day.

Some months after Lyn's funeral, I told Sarah and Kelly that I wanted them to have those rings to wear themselves as, purely coincidentally, emeralds and sapphires were their birth stones. I could not bear to think of them just sitting in a jewellery box, so I had them resized and Sarah and Kelly now wear them all the time—exactly what Lyn would have wanted.

I also had Lyn's wedding ring, a small heart-shaped locket and crucifix that she always wore made into a piece of jewellery on a neck chain, which I wear every day.

She always loved butterflies and would often wear a butterfly brooch, so now I wear that too.

Coming home

During the last couple of years, like many other people, I have researched my family tree online with Ancestry. I had traced some of my family, not to any great extent, but eighteen months ago I spent a long weekend with my cousin, Linda, in Derby. I had not seen her for twenty years, although we had kept in touch by email and phone.

Linda had done much more research on Ancestry than I had, and had traced her family back through several generations. We are second cousins; my mum, Winnie, had two half-sisters, Agnes and Emma; they had the same mother but different fathers.

Linda had traced our common eight times great-grandfather, William Bowden, back to 1605, when he was born in a village called Oakford. Coincidentally, it is ten minutes' drive from where I live now, so by moving here I have come full circle, back to my roots. I have since learned that his father, Willus Bowden, married Austice Maunder in 1600 in neighbouring Stoodleigh.

To date I have also traced some other branches of my family back to the mid-18th century.

48 Epilogue

Lyn and I were very fortunate to have quite a few relatives, lifelong friends and other friends whom we met along the way. We were both great believers in fate and that things happen and you meet people for a reason; those people were always there for us, for which Lyn and I were eternally grateful.

Lyn was always passionate about our family and our friends came a very close second. Keeping in touch with friends, in terms of telephoning, messaging, emailing and using WhatsApp, for example, is quite easy and more so in recent years. Keeping in touch with friends by meeting them can be more difficult when you are a full-time carer and feel you cannot leave your spouse, without them being cared for.

This did happen to me and I was limited as to whom I could visit, as well as where and how I could manage it, and for how long; not an easy thing to resolve.

Since Lyn's passing, I have kept in touch with my brother, Keith, his wife, Linda, and their children, Nicola and Daniel, also Lyn's brother Peter, his partner Kay, and their children, Amy and Christian, and Lyn's brother Neil's widow, Pik Lin. I have managed to visit my cousin, John, his wife, Fiona, and their daughter, Emma, as well as my cousins Susan, Linda, her son David and his partner Liam, with whom I kept in touch but had not seen for many years. I have also kept in touch with and visited Lyn's Welsh relatives, Marlene, and her daughters, Maia and Claire. Although I am English and proud of it, Lyn's

Welsh relatives adopted me long ago and I am proud of that too.

I have also visited Chrissie and Tim in France a couple of times; they retired a couple of years ago to a cottage in the same area as the farm. We have always kept in touch but it has been great to visit them and catch up.

We also had mutual close friends, who, over the years, effectively became family to Lyn, me and our daughters, and I continue see them. I have also been fortunate enough to catch up with many friends from my late teens, Tony, Andy, Michael, David, Gareth, John, Jack, Chris and Peter, with some of whom I have always kept in touch, with others not for some time, while their mutual friendship has continued. During the past two years, we have been able to meet in person, mainly every few months in London, close to where most of them are still based, for a few beers and a curry, which has been great fun. They all know about my life with Lyn and feel my pain and sorrow; they are always there for me but the banter, and all that goes with it, keeps me grounded. It reinforces the reasons why we became friends all those years ago; these have not changed and, when we get back together, it feels as if we are just catching up from yesterday. It is no different; we just have greyer hair—and less of it.

Maintaining friendships is incredibly important, even when it is not possible to meet in person, for whatever reason. There are so many ways of keeping in touch and I would always encourage people to do just that.

I have always supported the MS Society, and will continue to do so, in whatever way I can, such as raising awareness or fundraising, as the society helped us so much over the years. It is one of the reasons for writing this book.

Another reason is that, following Lyn's initial diagnosis, she was consistently supported by the NHS, local GPs, MS consultants, MS specialist nurses, physiotherapists and neuro-physiotherapists; they too deserve a mention.

I never thought that at some point in my life I would be sitting here in the evenings on my own, thinking about the loss of the love of my life. We think we are going to carry on forever. With Lyn's MS progressing, I always subconsciously accepted that the road we would travel together would not be a long one, but we have to put these thoughts out of our conscious minds and try to get on with life. If we do not, it eats away at us and we cannot support our wife or partner in the way we need to. Little did I know that something even worse would manifest itself and shorten the time that we had together.

We loved each other from almost as soon as we met and that love never stopped; if anything, it grew over time and we had forty-seven wonderful years together, through good and bad times.

I have also lost my best friend. I miss the times we shared, the times we talked and cried together, most of all the times we laughed together, which was very often; we always found something to laugh about, even on the darkest days.

When the girls were growing up, they said I was their rock; now Sarah and Steve, Kelly and Keith, and my grandchildren, Matt, Will, Hayden and Bethany, are my rocks and I know they are always there for me.

Live for the day; enjoy and cherish every single second because you will never get that chance again.

Live, love, and have no regrets.

*****

Lyn did not have a bad bone in her body and she had a huge heart; she was a beautiful woman, with a beautiful soul. Lyn abhorred any kind of upset, violence or fighting so I will end with her view on life, which she voiced throughout her life: 'Everybody should just love everybody.'

If only that were true, the world would be a far better place. Those simple words and this book are your legacy, my love.

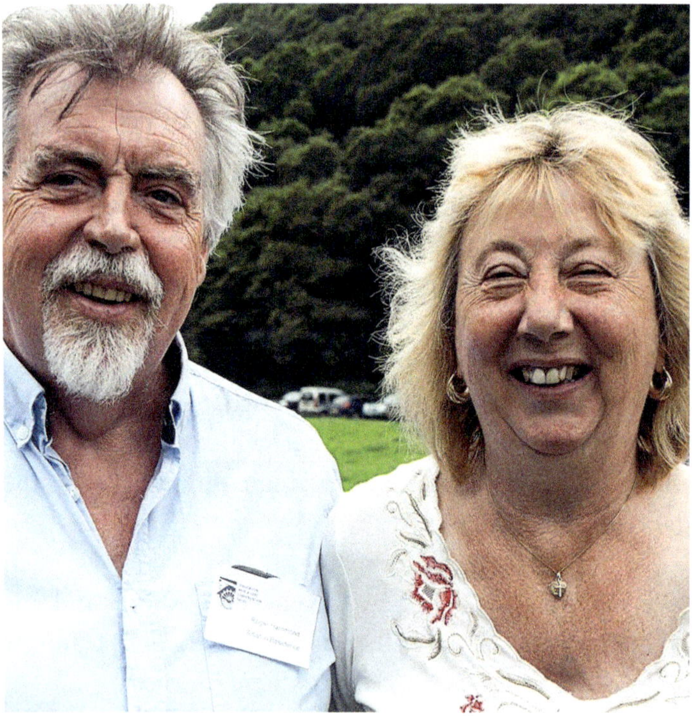

Lyn and me.

Acknowledgements

After I had started writing this book and, indeed, almost finished it, I started to look at ways of getting it published. I talked to a friend who was involved in publishing; he sent the initial draft to a literary agent, who said it was a good read but, due to the subject matter and the fact that I was completely unknown, it would be very difficult to place it with a publishing house.

I looked online to see how I could convert the manuscript to book format and then how to self publish. There were so many options, so I emailed a friend, Claire Savill, who, with Ceri Keene, is co-editor and publisher of our local bi-monthly magazine, *Exmoor News*. She replied almost immediately: 'You do know that we have published twenty-seven books to date?'

'No, I didn't know! Can we meet up to talk about it?'

So I have to thank Claire and Ceri for their invaluable help in enabling me to have this book published. I also have to thank Diane Trembath for doing the initial and subsequent copy editing of each draft, as the book's contents expanded or its structure changed, and for keeping me on the straight and narrow with the essentials, such as correct punctuation and syntax. Publishing would not have been possible without their help.

Thanks to my friend, Professor John Greenwood, who kindly looked at the original draft and made some very astute observations, which I have included.

In a conversation about the book, my friend, Michael

Messer, suggested that it might be best if I softened the title to avoid it being perceived as a medical treatise about MS. This was good advice.

A big thank you to my daughters, Sarah and Kelly, who were the first readers of the initial draft. It was important to have their approval for what I was proposing, and I was grateful for their continued support and encouragement, as there were times when I wondered if I was doing the right thing. Whenever I doubted what I was doing, something would happen, or support would come from an unexpected direction, which then made me realise that I should finish what I had set out to do.

Photo acknowledgements

All photographs included in this book have been taken by the author or are from his collection except: photo Australia outback ballooning, by permission of Outback Ballooning, Alice Springs, Australia.

Sources of Information

MS Society
Carriage House
8 City North Place
London N4 3FU
tel: 0808 800 800
www.mssociety.org.uk
For anyone affected by MS, including patients, carers and families—includes information on research, community, services and support.

NHS England
www.nhs.uk/conditions/multiple-sclerosis/
General healthcare information and services, including MS symptoms, diagnosis and treatment.

The Motability Scheme is run by Motability Operations Ltd
22 Bishopsgate
London EC2N 4BQ
www.motability.co.uk

Blue Badge Scheme
www.gov.uk/apply-blue-badge

Harrow MS Therapy Centre
Harrow School Farm
Watford Road
Harrow HA1 3TS
tel: 020 8423 6268
www.harrowmscentre.co.uk

South West MS Therapy Centre
West Grange
Clyst Heath
Exeter EX2 7EY
tel: 01392 447411
www.southwestmscentre.co.uk
There are MS Therapy Centres around the country, check local availability.

Citizens Advice Centre
www.citizensadvice.org.uk
There are Citizens Advice Centres around the country; check local availability.

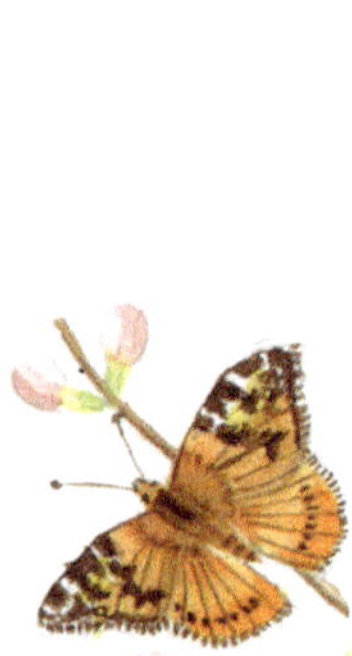

Printed in Dunstable, United Kingdom

71521479R10167